Pink for a Girl

Pink for a Girl

Wanting a baby and not conceiving – my personal story

Isla McGuckin

HAY HOUSE

HAY HOUSE
Australia • Canada • Hong Kong
South Africa • United Kingdom • United States

First published and distributed in the United Kingdom by
Hay House UK Ltd, Unit 62, Canalot Studios,
222 Kensal Rd, London W10 5BN.
Tel.: (44) 20 8962 1230; Fax: (44) 20 8962 1239.
www.hayhouse.co.uk

Published and distributed in the United States of America by
Hay House, Inc., PO Box 5100, Carlsbad, CA 92018-5100.
Tel: (1) 760 431 7695 or (800) 654 5126;
Fax (1) 760 431 6948 or (800) 650 5115.
www.hayhouse.com

Published and distributed in Australia by
Hay House Australia Ltd, 18/36 Ralph St, Alexandra NSW 2015.
Tel: (61) 2 9669 4299; Fax: (61) 2 9669 4144.
www.hayhouse.com.au

Published and distributed in the Republic of South Africa by
Hay House SA (Pty), Ltd, PO Box 990, Witkoppen 2068.
Tel./Fax: (27) 11 706 6612. orders@psdprom.co.za

Distributed in Canada by
Raincoast, 9050 Shaughnessy St, Vancouver, BC V6P 6E5.
Tel: (1) 604 323 7100; Fax: (1) 604 323 2600

© Isla McGuckin, 2006

A catalogue record for this book is available from the British Library.

ISBN 1-4019-0743-1

Design: Leanne Siu
Typesetting: Peter Powell Origination & Print Limited

Printed and bound in Great Britain by
TJ International, Padstow, Cornwall

For Paul,
and for the children I would have chosen for myself:
Amber, Fred, Gabriel, Millie, Genevieve, Callum, Poppy,
Freya, Phoebe, Ben.

Foreword

Couples experiencing fertility problems often feel very alone and can find it difficult to articulate their fears and their concerns. Pink for a Girl will help to promote discussion between partners who are finding it difficult to name their feelings surrounding their own infertility. Pink for a Girl will also prove invaluable for the friends and the families, the doctors and the therapists of those couples who are experiencing fertility problems; people who may otherwise have no idea of the depth and complexity of the emotions surrounding the issue.

Introduction

I am not a doctor.

I am not an alternative practitioner.

I am not a fertility expert.

In fact, I am not any kind of an expert.

But I do know what it's like to want to have children and not be able to have them.

And I do know what it's like to feel left behind as friend after friend after friend announces their 'happy news'.

And I do know what it's like to want to have a baby so badly that, sometimes, it hurts.

And I do know what it's like to feel as though time and options and hope are running out.

Don't worry, though. My story isn't all doom and gloom. It even has a happy ending. Just not the happy ending – that I'd been expecting.

Pink for a Girl is *my* story. It is a story about the incredible sadness of involuntary childlessness, but it's also a story about the indestructibility of human spirit and of hope.

Isla McGuckin

Our 'Some-Time-in-the-Future' Baby

We had managed to escape to Australia for a whole month. Just the two of us, chilling on a deserted Cairns beach, soaking up the very last of the day's sun and reliving the highlight of our holiday so far, a trip to the Great Barrier Reef. A trip that had been awe-inspiring and cliché-inducing; a trip that had been humbling, somehow; a trip where we had both appreciated just what tiny components we were, as human beings, in 'The Great Scheme of Things'.

And rather lazily, rather languidly – we carried on talking. Just a stream of consciousness, really, our thoughts made fluid by our day in the sun. We talked about the still brand new millennium. We talked about life, the universe and where the two of us fitted into it all. We had always known that we fitted together. Isla and Paul. Paul and Isla. Together forever. That was a given. For both of us. Passers-by could have easily mistaken us for honeymooners, as we lay there on that beautiful beach, in the soft early evening light. Our beach towels were lying so close together that they almost overlapped, our his 'n' hers airport paperbacks were face down in the sand, long since forgotten, both of us far more interested in each other than in the plot of any novel. Because even though we had been married for more than five years by then, we still seemed to have so much to talk about.

And on that languorous and sun-soaked day – on the eve of my twenty-ninth birthday, our conversation worked its way around to the subject of children. And we talked about the possibility of us having them. Some of our friends had already started to have babies; some already had a couple. And, although we loved to look after our friends' children for a few hours or for an evening, up until that point we had both always been quite happy to hand those kids back to their parents at the end of the day. Glad to get back to our life of relative freedom. Glad to get back to a life that was unencumbered by sleepless nights and by potty training, by bedtime routines and by temper tantrums. Both of us had always wanted to have kids though. We had both wanted to have a family *eventually*, some time in the future. In fact, we had said as much before we had even got together, when we were 'just good friends'. But until that lazy day on the beach in Oz, there had always seemed to be more questions than answers, for us, about the 'having-a-baby' issue.

Would we be good parents? Would we be *good enough* parents? Were we ready for the responsibility of a tiny human being relying on us for absolutely everything? Had we grown up enough yet ourselves? How would we feel about putting our social life on hold for a year (or for five years, or for ten years, or for twenty years)? Would I ever be able to get into a pair of size ten jeans again? What about spending hours in the bath, smothered in beauty treatments, sipping white wine and leafing through glossy magazines? Shallow as a teaspoon, I know, but still … And how would our relationship be affected?

Would we have any energy left for each other after disturbed nights and feeding on demand? Would Paul still fancy me after watching me give birth? Come to think of it, after giving birth, would I ever even *want* him to fancy me again? What about our careers? Were we stable enough financially to have a baby? Could we cope with such a huge drop in income? Would I be able to, or want to, pick up where I left off after maternity leave? Would Paul feel overwhelmed by financial responsibility? Pressurized into being the sole breadwinner? Was our house big enough? Was it child-friendly enough? Was it in the right catchment area for the best possible local schools …?

And maybe because we *were* lying on that far-flung beach, a million miles away from the puzzling practicalities of potential parenthood, we realized that we were as ready as we were ever going to be for our 'some-time-in-the-future' baby. And, as scarily life-changing as having a baby appeared to be, Paul and I realized that we were both happy for 'some time in the future' to be sooner rather than later.

'Just Have Lots and Lots of Fun!'

As soon as we got home from our trip, I made an appointment with the nurse at our local health centre to check out one or two baby making facts. I may have been just a year away from thirty and, as a woman, I was aware that I was probably supposed to have that kind of knowledge innately. But I wanted someone to tell me – and I wanted that someone to be medical and official and, well, grown-up and responsible – whether making a baby really was as straightforward as just chucking away my contraceptive pills and letting nature take its course.

I remember taking a seat in the health centre's crowded waiting room and experiencing the same sense of nervous apprehension that I had done many years before while I was waiting for the oral bit of my French 'O' level. I ran through likely scenarios in my mind. I mentally rehearsed what I was going to say. I deliberated about how to phrase my questions. The only difference was that, instead of feeling anxious about the prospect of having to re-sit my French 'O' level, I was worried that I was going to appear – and to someone authoritative, to a health care professional – as though I was someone who was too dim-witted to even contemplate a pregnancy.

'What lovely news!' the practice nurse had exclaimed, when my turn finally came round and I had managed to ineloquently blurt out my query, 'Now, just throw one lot of pills away and replace them with some new ones!'

'Folic acid, silly,' she had giggled – somewhat patronizingly as I recall – in response to my rather bemused expression, 'Now you just go away and make sure that you and your partner have lots and lots of fun!'

And nine short and 'lots and lots of fun' filled months later, the stork delivered a special little bundle, just for Paul and me …

Hmm. I suppose it would be nice if real life actually worked out like that, once in a while. But the reality was, *twelve* months later, the lots and lots of fun that had been prescribed for us was, gradually, starting to be replaced by lots and lots of doubt. And I remember wondering just how long it was supposed to take, getting pregnant. Was it one month? Was it six months? A year? And I remember acknowledging that by the time the doubt had set in, I had celebrated my thirtieth birthday and so a full year had already been and gone. And I remember thinking that surely *something* should have happened, in that length of time.

On the beach in Australia, all those months before, when Paul and I had made the decision to start trying for our baby, we had also made the decision that trying for a baby would be our little secret. That we would keep to ourselves until we had something to actually *tell* people. But, with the passing of that disappointingly uneventful year, I made up my mind to re-think that decision. I decided to break our self-imposed code of silence so that I could get some more advice, to supplement what the nurse at our local health centre had told me. I decided to have a quiet word with one of my friends, a friend with two kids who obviously knew something that I didn't.

The Right (and Wrong) Time of the Month

'Well, are you sure that you're doing it at the right time of the month?'

'Eh?' It was obvious that my friend with two kids *did* know something that I didn't. Even now, I can remember being taken aback by the irony of it all. Taken aback by the irony that in a so-called developed nation and in the twenty-first century – the *information* age, for goodness sake – a university-educated woman like me should know so very little about her own body. And what a waste it was, in hindsight, of all of those (evidently pointless) anxious days spent by teenage girls, the world over, waiting, fingers-crossed, for a period to start. Those schoolyard horror stories that had seemed to be rife in my youth – and that had probably been instigated by over-protective parents who should have known better – about girls getting pregnant *without even having* sex certainly had a lot to answer for.

I think I had pictured myself as some kind of super-fertile deity of womanhood, just waiting to start popping my babies out by the dozen, as soon as I had decided that the time was right. And although I probably did have some sort of vague notion about fertile days, could I really have been the only wannabe mother who didn't find out till the age of thirty that women only get a conception window of a measly couple of days each month? And, with this newly acquired information in mind, what was the point of taking contraceptive pills for twenty-one days out of twenty-eight? Now that seemed to me to be as perfect an example of overkill as you could ever hope to hear.

And with the conception window revelation, it seemed that my friend had just been warming up. It seemed that she had even more pearls of baby making wisdom to share with me.

'It isn't just the timing that has to be right either, you know. You've got to be in the right frame of mind. Focused but not obsessive, relaxed but receptive,' my friend paused for dramatic effect before she continued, '*and* you need to be in the right position, sexually. You need to be in the missionary position, ideally, and have your bum elevated by pillows and your legs raised for a good half an hour after the event to help the little tadpoles on their way.'

'Hang on a minute! Are you going to make this baby making business sound any less romantic? Are you going to make this baby making business sound any less *fun*?'

And even as those indignant words came tumbling out of my mouth I remember thinking that, presumably for *optimum* baby making results, you really did need to be in the same country as your partner during each month's paltry couple of fertile days, too.

I was working for the UK division of a large, international food manufacturing company when Paul and I had made the decision to knock our chosen method of contraception on the head and see what happened. My role in that company's marketing department had called for lots of cross-divisional meetings with local production teams and local sales teams and so, consequently, I needed to travel extensively and regularly throughout Europe. I suppose that the *idea* of it all sounds pretty glamorous and, in lots of ways, the reality of it all was pretty glamorous to with business class flights and gorgeous hotels and generous expense accounts. But it seems that overseas business meetings are far from ideal when you and your partner are trying to have a baby.

I remember grabbing my diary out of my bag and flicking through its pages as I mentally calculated the fertile days in my last few cycles. I registered the sheer volume of appointments of international business trips, of overseas team meetings – and I quickly lost count of the number of occasions when the optimum day for baby making nookie, for Paul and me, had also frustratingly coincided with the middle of a week-long tour of Scandinavia. And then I must have blurted out my initial thoughts, my knee-jerk reaction to the situation, because I noticed that my friend was looking at me as though I had lost the plot.

'What? I'm just asking the question. Do you think that it's *physically* possible?'

'To take a sealed Tupperware container – suitably and freshly filled – and a turkey baster with you in your hand luggage? And then to use them, on your fertile days, on your business trips, to get yourself pregnant?'

'Yeah.'

'And five minutes ago, you were complaining about the *missionary position* being unromantic! No, I don't think that it's physically possible. And I don't think that it's particularly sane either.'

I knew it. And, as far as I was aware, *virtual* conception was still not a medical possibility at that stage either. And so that was it. My spectacularly badly-timed, once-monthly European team meetings were going to have to go.

Working (and Hoping-to-Be) Mother

It was like taking on another project at work and a highly confidential one at that. Trying surreptitiously to take a step back from my career and making excuses to avoid as many international meetings as possible, without looking like I was some kind of work-shy slacker who really didn't deserve their industry-competitive salary or their company car, their generous benefits package or their final salary pension scheme. But I persevered as best I could. Keeping up the *appearance* of commitment at work, while making a conscious effort to be within grabbing distance of Paul on my fertile days.

I had switched companies enough times, during my ten years of mostly gainful employment, to pull together what seemed like a fairly representative picture of just how negatively pregnant women could be perceived in the workplace. I had witnessed mothers-to-be being treated incredibly dismissively, as though they were just a baby step away from being imbeciles, as though the only things that they could put their minds to were birthing plans and nursery colour schemes. And I had noticed that there had often seemed to be an undercurrent of quite bitter resentment towards them – from both male *and* female colleagues. There seemed to be a sense that pregnant women had somehow let the side down. A sense that they had somehow been disloyal; cold-heartedly adding to their stressed out colleagues' workloads while *they* were able to swan about on maternity leave for anything up to a year.

And I had heard plenty of horror stories about working mums too. I had heard about them attempting to squeeze a full-time job into part-time hours and for part-time pay. I had heard about them being overlooked for promotions because their true commitment 'obviously' lay elsewhere. I had heard about them being first in line for redundancy because they just didn't cut it any more. When it came to working mothers, the tales of injustice just seemed to go on and on. I really couldn't face putting myself through all of that, certainly not before I had even managed to get pregnant.

But it wasn't easy, keeping mum about trying to become a mum. I remember getting the feeling that some of my work colleagues, the ones that I was closest to, the ones with whom I spent the most time, were already starting to get suspicious. I had always had a reputation at work for being highly organized and as ambitious as the next woman; for being one of the first to volunteer their services for any high profile, overseas projects. But suddenly, and in a way that was completely out of character, there I was. Double booking myself left, right and centre and making anything UK-based my top priority just so that I could avoid being away from home at those crucial-for-conception moments.

However, despite my newly absorbing preoccupation with juggling my diary and with re-prioritizing my workload, I had become aware of a nagging little voice. And although the little voice was right at the back of my mind, I couldn't quite ignore it; no matter how hard I tried. The little voice kept telling me that maybe I needed to face up to the facts. Maybe I couldn't really afford to be damaging my career prospects. Maybe a high-flying and work-focused future was going to be my *only* future. No matter what else I hoped for, no matter what else I dreamed about. And, as the months passed, that nagging little voice became louder and even more persistent. It was fuelled by colleague pregnancy announcement after colleague pregnancy announcement. And, as my fourth colleague in as many weeks announced that they, or their wife, their girlfriend or some random stranger that they had shagged once in a pub car park was pregnant, I found that it was virtually impossible to maintain my professionalism, my sense of composure. I found that it was all that I could do to restrain myself from shouting, 'You lucky, lucky bastard!' and flouncing out of whichever office I had the misfortune of being in.

The Great Conception Conspiracy

'Am I the only woman, in the entire bloody world, who didn't get pregnant the first month of trying?' The trying-for-a-baby code of silence well and truly broken amongst our nearest and dearest, this was me, opening yet another conversation with yet another newly pregnant friend with the only topic that seemed to be of any interest to me.

'Everyone else that I speak to is like, "Oh, I'd only just come off the pill" or, "Yes, it *is* a bit of a surprise, but we are both very happy about it" or, "We forgot to use a condom one night and – bingo!"'

'Well, we were trying for six months before I got pregnant. At least six months, actually. In fact, it was probably more like eight months.'

'But, you said …'

'I know I did, I know. Don't ask me why.'

'I *will* ask you why. *Why?*'

'I guess we just didn't want to tell people that we were trying for a baby in case nothing happened. And then when something eventually *did* happen, when I got pregnant ... Well, what was the point of telling people that we'd spent eight months thinking the worst?'

Hmm. To ease the poor, tortured minds of your friends, maybe? To ease the poor, tortured minds of women like me who were struggling to reassure themselves that they didn't have anything to worry about in the baby making department? But I also knew that if I was being one hundred per cent honest I probably – all right, *definitely* – would have done exactly the same thing as my friend. Paul and I had been trying for our baby for well over a year before I had even *mentioned* the fact to my very closest friends. And I had only spoken to them then because I needed their help and wanted their advice.

There is a sort of competitiveness about conception that I had never realized existed before, a sort of 'look how fertile I am' one-upmanship. And all that one-upmanship does is to perpetuate the myth that it's easy, getting pregnant, that there really is nothing to it. And so I decided to check out the facts. I decided to do a bit of research in an attempt to reassure myself, in an attempt to put my *own* mind at rest. I checked out a few of the more reliable-looking websites and I discovered that it takes the average late twenties, early thirties couple *at least* six to twelve months to conceive. And so it seemed that the vast majority of people for whom 'it just happened' must either have been super-fertile freaks of nature or big fat liars.

Complications – His

Maybe the conception-competitiveness, the 'look how fertile I am' one-upmanship had started to get the better of us. Maybe Paul and I had been trying a bit *too* hard for that rather elusive baby of ours. Out of the blue, Paul had started to suffer from severe pain in his groin, combined – rather worryingly – with a bout of debilitating dizzy spells. When Paul made an appointment with his GP to get himself checked out, his doctor was blunt with his diagnosis, and to the point, in the inimitable style of a true Yorkshire-man.

'You've ruptured yourself, lad.'

A hernia. But happily, as it turned out, a hernia that was completely unrelated to our trying, no matter how vigorously, for our baby. We both thanked our lucky stars for my company's private medical insurance scheme when we realized that an op was going to be needed to fix 'the rupture'. And by going privately, we managed to bypass the usual six-month waiting list and Paul had an appointment with the hernia consultant before the week of his diagnosis was out.

Poor Paul. For him, that appointment with the hernia consultant kicked off a month-long programme of ignominy and discomfort. And it started straightaway, in the consultant's examination room, where I had tagged along to provide Paul with some moral support. The consultant had asked Paul to drop his trousers so that he could get a good look at the hernia. And then the consultant had shot me a lewd wink before asking, 'Is that as big as it gets?' Paul had had his back to me, but I could see the cheeks of his bottom flush pink and I could only assume that the ones on his face were doing the same.

And, for Paul, it seemed that the very worst of the humiliation was still to come. Little more than a week after his initial appointment with the hernia consultant, Paul had been installed in a hospital bed, in a private room. He was doing the best that he could, under the circumstances, to make himself comfortable. He started to look distinctly *uncomfortable*, though, when a camp and yet butch-looking man who was sporting an impressively stereotypical handlebar moustache knocked on his bedroom door. Paul had started to look positively panic-stricken when he registered that the man was carrying a pretty serious looking cutthroat razor on a gleaming stainless steel tray. It seemed that Freddie Mercury's body double had arrived to give Paul his pre-op Brazilian.

A week after what had, in the end, turned out to be a textbook successful hernia repair operation and on the morning of his birthday, of all days, Paul had one final appointment. An appointment with the nurse at our local health centre; it was time for the last stage in his hernia repair process; it was time for Paul's stitches to be removed. Now, come on, do birthday treats *get* any better than that?

En route to the health centre, we checked our mailbox for birthday cards for Paul and we retrieved a fairly official-looking brown envelope addressed to me, too. I tore the envelope open, skimming over its contents as we walked along the drive to our car, thoroughly expecting to be reading about yet another once-in-a-lifetime prize draw opportunity for lucky Mrs McGuckin. But, instead, the contents of that brown envelope made my heart lurch and I started to feel decidedly sick. After more than ten years of trouble-free cervical smears, I had been recalled.

Complications – Hers

I remember thinking that at least we were heading to the health centre; surely that was a better destination than most to get some answers to the questions that had already started to buzz around in my head. And so, while Paul was otherwise engaged with the practice nurse, I managed to collar my doctor for an unscheduled appointment between her other appointments. And I remember feeling grateful for that, knowing that it was no mean feat in these times of over-worked and under-resourced NHS GPs.

'Mmm. The suggestion of severe dyskariosis,' my doctor read out the relevant section from my medical notes.

Now, the suggestion of anything that was unpronounceable by the layman had always been enough to send me into a blind panic and so the rest of the conversation largely washed over me. I tried hard to concentrate on what my doctor was saying to me. I tried hard to control my thoughts as they leapt and darted and jumped to conclusions. But, in the end, the only fact that I managed to glean was the one that told me that I needed to make an appointment with a gynaecologist up at the hospital – an appointment for an investigative procedure, for something called a colposcopy. Then, as soon as I saw the opportunity, I made a bolt for it, back to the relative refuge of the waiting room. Once there, I sank rather dispiritedly into a plastic chair that was still warm from the bottom of its previous occupant and tried to lose myself in an article about easy summer entertaining – it was November – while I waited for Paul.

Later that night, I headed out for fish and chips. Paul was still far from ready for a big night out to celebrate his birthday but both of us needed some kind of treat – no matter how small that treat was – after the joyless day that we had just had to endure. On my way home from the chip shop, in an attempt to drown out the choir of negativity that had been relentless in my head since my informal little chat with my doctor – a chorus of concern about just what exactly an abnormal smear could imply – I switched on my car stereo. It wasn't the greatest of moves. A song from the *Moulin Rouge* soundtrack was playing, a cover version of *'One Day I'll Fly Away'*. Every lyric of every line seemed to strike a chord with me until I was completely awash with self pity and my tears became so torrential that I had to pull over to compose myself; ever mindful of the fish and chips that were growing cold and congealing greasily in their newspaper beside me.

I had to remind myself that Paul's list of birthday goodies had so far included: the painful removal of stitches from a fairly major operation that he was still less than 50 per cent recovered from, the discovery that I needed some quite serious sounding gynaecological examinations, and the prospect of a less than fun-filled night in front of a distinctly midweek TV schedule. Accompanied by (the now cold) fish and chips. I knew that Paul could really do without a hysterical wife to add to that unhappy trinity. So I pulled myself together and slowly made my way home.

Complications – More of the Bloody Things

Slowly but surely, the weeks passed – as weeks, eventually, always do – and my hot date with the gynaecologist arrived. I had been reliably informed that a colposcopy was basically just a more in-depth version of a smear, that a colposcopy was nothing at all to worry about. Well, you can call me a stress-bunny, but having your legs in stirrups and your vulnerability exposed and magnified onto a TV screen beside you, with a trolley chock-full of medical equipment strongly resembling mediaeval instruments of torture waiting and glinting, evilly and metallically, in the harsh light of a hospital surgery, certainly seemed like something to worry about to me.

The nurse quickly picked up on the abject terror that was threatening to engulf me while I waited for her and the gynae-cologist to complete their pre-colposcopy preparations. And so she did her best to reassure me, to comfort me. She held my hand throughout the entire, rather grim, procedure. She urged me to concentrate on my breathing. She recommended that I really should start to exhale or I would run the risk of passing out. And she told me, in what I remember thinking was an inappropriately cheerful fashion, that 'some ladies prefer to watch on screen.'

And so I did as she had suggested. I watched on screen. And despite watching on screen making the whole procedure seem a hundred times worse and, surely, a hundred times bigger, I found that I was unable to tear my eyes away. God, what is wrong with me? I remember thinking. And why would anyone want to watch *that*? Every time the gynaecologist probed, I could see (and, of course, feel) everything. I started to worry that I had developed masochistic tendencies to add to my current batch of troubles. And I realized that I really did need to exhale.

What couldn't have been much more than ten minutes later – although it certainly felt more like ten *hours* – the colposcopy was over. But unfortunately for me, that wasn't quite the end of the procedure. The colposcopy had revealed that I needed to book myself in for a session of treatment to get rid of the rogue cells that had been discovered. I needed a type of treatment called cold coagulation, a treatment that sounded almost as unpleasant as it actually turned out to be. Cold coagulation was a cross between laser treatment and freezing and it left me with painful, period-type cramps for several days afterwards. But as unpleasant as those cramps were, they were a walk in the park compared to the other side effect that I experienced: vile-smelling, watery and profuse vaginal discharge that seemed to continue for weeks afterwards. Nice.

Another colposcopy – I must admit that it seemed like an absolute breeze after my experience with cold coagulation – and a couple more smears later and I finally got the all clear. And I could concentrate, once more, on trying to get pregnant.

Excuses, Excuses ...

And so we had been given the all clear on both counts. Paul was fully recovered from his hernia repair operation and my cervical smear results were back to normal. I had been off the pill for what was getting close to two years and I had been enlightened about the concept of fertile days for almost a year. But still, whenever Paul and I started talking about our lack-of-baby situation, I just couldn't stop myself from making excuses for us. I guess that a therapist would have called it denial.

'Well I suppose that we were out of action from a baby making point of view – for a couple of months, at least, after your hernia op.'

'Not exactly – I can vividly recall you diving on me the day before I had my stitches out because it was "the right time".'

'Well, maybe I've been travelling too much again, then. Maybe, because of that, we've missed more opportunities than we've realized.'

'Hardly. You plan our months with almost military precision these days. And, anyway, you hardly ever do any travelling any more.'

I remember pausing, searching for another straw that I could clutch at, 'I guess that all of that business with my abnormal smears can't have helped ...'

'No, your doctor *and* your gynaecologist told you that there wasn't really a link there.'

'Oh, come on Paul. Let me have just one bloody glimmer of hope to cling to, please! I don't think I can cope, knowing that I've been off the pill for two years and that we've been shagging at the right time of the month for at least one year and that *still* nothing's happened!'

I paused again, before taking a deep breath, before blurting out something that I think we had both been secretly suspecting for months, 'There's got to be something wrong with one of us, hasn't there?'

The Green-Eyed Monster

By that stage, two of my very closest friends had already had kids. And, despite the fact that one of those friends had conceived their second child when Paul and I had been trying for our baby for over a year, that was OK. Both of us were all right with that. Maybe because when that particular couple had *started* their baby making, baby making still wasn't really on the agenda for Paul and me.

There had been so many other things that we had wanted to do first, while we still had the opportunity, before kids came along. Both of us had wanted to travel, for a start. We had wanted to see the world. We had wanted to enjoy some quality time together. We had wanted to blow some of our hard-earned cash in some exotic and far-flung places. We had wanted to have an adventure or two, something to tell the grandchildren. And there was a long list of more everyday, mundane things that Paul and I had wanted to get out of the way, too. We had wanted to clear our student debts, to pay off the overdrafts and the credit card bills. We had wanted to *use* our degrees, to get decent jobs, to climb up a few rungs of the career ladder. We had wanted to bag ourselves a little bit of financial security – to buy a house, to save up a little nest egg for ourselves and for our 'some-time-in-the-future' baby.

But then I guessed – correctly as it turned out, too many uncharacteristically sober nights out had been a dead give-away – that a different close friend was pregnant with her *first* child. And somehow – inexplicably – that *wasn't* OK.

I felt as though I was completely out of control of my emotions as they lurched from one extreme to another. Rationally, I was happy for my friend, of course I was. I knew that she and her husband hadn't had it easy either; that they had both begun to question their fertility after trying for a baby for a while, without success. And morally, of course, I knew that it would be very wrong of me to wish infertility on someone else – to wish infertility on one of my closest friends – just because that was what seemed to be facing Paul and me. But I was also insanely jealous. And I had never experienced anything like it before. Not even when a classmate's starting salary after university was more than double the pittance of a pay packet that I had managed to negotiate for myself. Not even when one of my bosses had got themselves a shiny new company car while I was still struggling to work in an unreliable and un-roadworthy heap of rusting metal. Not even when a friend had got engaged while I was rather painfully trying to extricate myself from a relationship that was way past its use-by date.

Somehow, this jealousy felt different. It felt raw and desperate, it felt primal and it felt real. Why wasn't it *our* turn to have a baby? Why did *we* have to be the ones who found getting pregnant to be such a struggle? If it was true that five out of six couples managed to conceive without medical help, then why did Paul and I have to be the sixth? And why, oh why, didn't I keep my big mouth shut? Why didn't I keep my top conception tips to myself?

I started to become aware of quite a sharp and vivid sense of fear. I was afraid of being left behind. I was frightened that if Paul and I never managed to have a baby of our own we would eventually have less and, ultimately, nothing in common with our friends, as baby after baby, of theirs, came along. And other people's babies – other friends' babies – just seemed to keep on coming. I could see our life changing beyond recognition and beyond my control. I imagined that the social life of our future would be more about toddler-friendly picnics than big nights out. I imagined that our conversations would have to be sanitized and U-rated because you never knew which little angel was within earshot. And, scarier still, I imagined that ultimately Paul and I were going to be excluded from a cosy little club to which we so desperately wanted to belong. I pictured a middle-aged couple, sozzled, propping up a bar, drinking together to drown their sorrows, oblivious to the sniggers of the groups of teens and twenty-somethings that surrounded them. I pictured that middle-aged couple with my face and Paul's …

And I started to get the distinct impression that sympathy had a shelf life, too. Friends were as kind as their patience allowed. They did their best not to glaze over when I launched into yet another tirade bemoaning the unfairness of my inability to conceive. They tried to understand where I was coming from when I complained about the dark cloud of involuntary childlessness that seemed to be hanging over Paul and me. But I knew that, eventually, I was going to have to put up or shut up. Eventually, I was going to have to stop talking about infertility even though it was the single most important issue in my life and in Paul's. I knew that if I didn't, I would risk driving our friends away. And a future with neither babies nor friends seemed like one that was just far too painful to contemplate.

I knew that Paul and I needed to do something. The time had come to take action. And so we decided to bite the bullet and to get ourselves checked out. For the sake of our own sanity – and for that of our friends – we needed to find out why, after two years of contraception-free sex, there was still no baby McGuckin on the horizon.

Tadpole Testing

It was Paul who got the ball rolling (pun intended) but somewhat unofficially. Flicking through one of his usual lowbrow men's magazines one day, he had spotted a small classified ad promoting an in-home 'Tadpole Testing' kit. Hmm. Looking back, I am amazed that the whole tone of the thing hadn't alerted at least one of us to the likely inaccuracies of the test results. But in good faith, Paul had called the 'Tadpole Testing' hotline, passed over his credit card details and the Tadpole Test had arrived in the post just a couple of days later. Tadpole Testing, maybe not surprisingly, had turned out to be a pretty low-tech affair. Paul simply had to do the appropriate business into the receptacle provided and immerse into the receptacle a reactive paper strip. And then all that we had to do was to set our kitchen timer for the five minutes that the 'Tadpole Test' took to develop and await our fate.

'Gutted' is an understatement to describe how the pair of us felt that Friday evening when Paul failed the 'Tadpole Test'. I started to cry and then Paul did, too. We hugged each other as though the possibility of our 'some-time-in-the-future' baby becoming a reality depended on it. And then, as our tears gradually began to subside, we started to talk. Brave words just kept pouring out of both of our mouths.

We said that all that really mattered was that we were together. We said that all that really mattered was that we had each other. And we tentatively mooted adoption as an alternative. We said that maybe it didn't matter, not being able to have our own, biological kids. Maybe, by adopting, we could still have the family that we both so badly wanted. But no amount of brave words, no amount of fighting talk, could hide the fact that both of us were totally and utterly devastated. And so we set to work, attempting to drown our sorrows at the bottom of a couple of bottles of wine.

The alcohol therapy was ineffectual; it was a temporary fix at best. So the next day Paul and I decided that we would try to spend our way out of our gloominess and we headed into town for a spot of retail therapy. It was a mood-matching grey and overcast English winter's morning. In fact it was so grey and overcast that Paul decided to drive to town with his headlights on. Or, rather, *headlight*. We were about a mile from home, when we saw blue flashing lights behind us. 'Damn,' I remember thinking, 'They're going to pull us over.' Paul and I started frantically calculating units of alcohol and hours passed since consumed. And we pulled over.

'Did you check your headlights this morning, sir, like you're supposed to do every morning?'

It is always a dilemma, be honest and get yourself into really big style bother – 'Actually, it's all that I can do to remember to put the petrol in' – or fib. Just a little bit. Paul was asked to step into the police car that had pulled into the lay-by behind us and I had no choice but to wait, as patiently as I could. I waited for what seemed like an absolute eternity as every possible scenario and quite a few impossible ones played themselves out in my head. I became convinced that the police officer would breathalyze Paul. And that was one test that we really *didn't* want to be positive. And so I practically dislocated my neck, craning to see what was going on behind me, through the rear-view mirror. I thought that an obvious turn, to look over my shoulder, would look like an admission of guilt. That it would make me look like an accessory to whatever crime Paul was being accused of. As the minutes dragged past, my thoughts continued to descend into a spiral of absolute doom.

If the police officer *did* breathalyze Paul, he was bound to still be over the limit. It was sod's law. He would lose his licence. He would lose his job, for God's sake. He worked in sales and he was expected to be able to drive hundreds of miles, every single week. Oh my God, my husband would have a criminal record and for drunken driving. *Drunken driving*. That was almost as bad as attempted murder, in my book. We would never be approved for adoption if Paul had just got himself saddled with a criminal record for drunken driving …

Finally, Paul walked back up the lay-by toward our car. Alone. I couldn't work out, at first, whether that was a good thing or not.

'I've got a producer,' Paul told me, as he climbed back into the driver's seat.

'A what?'

'A producer – I've just got to take my documents down to the police station on Monday.'

'Thank you, God.'

Tadpole Testing – A Second Opinion

I really don't know why we had chosen to use such an unorthodox method for testing Paul's potency. I don't know why Paul hadn't just gone to his doctor in the first place. I guess that some of it was embarrassment. The prospect of delivering by hand a still warm sample pot to our local and usually jam-packed health centre was not a particularly appealing one for either of us. And I think that the rest of our reticence was down to fear. If a properly trained doctor had said that Paul was shooting blanks, then that was pretty much it. Ruling out sperm donation – and I think I can safely say that both of us would have done – our baby dreams would have been effectively over. Our worst fears would have been realized, and with medical authority.

Although I still don't really understand what most of the test results mean, I will never forget the sense of relief that I felt when Paul's *official* semen analysis report was returned to us. Millions of one thing and extremely high percentages of several others; it certainly seemed as though Paul had an awful lot of particularly strong swimmers. And Paul's doctor had been quick to confirm the good news. He had told us that, from a tadpole point of view, we really didn't have anything to worry about. And so that was that. Paul was OK and it was over to me. It was my turn to get checked out. If only the tests for female fertility were as straightforward as wanking into a sample pot.

Tadpole Testing – The Female Equivalent

I felt as though I was a young schoolgirl who had inadvertently stumbled into an advanced degree level lecture on the female reproductive system. As my doctor bombarded me with terms like follicle stimulating, gonadotropin releasing and luteinizing hormones, my eyes began to glaze over and my mind began to wander. The fact that any woman had ever managed to navigate such a complex and highly sensitive process successfully enough to become pregnant was beginning to seem like nothing short of a miracle to me.

The first step in the female equivalent of tadpole testing was to make sure that I was doing the ovulation bit of the conception process correctly. My doctor asked me to make another appointment, to time it for a mid(ish) cycle, for a blood test that would help her to do just that. My gynaecologist had already told me in between colposcopies and cold coagulation treatment that, despite being painful, my very regular periods were actually quite a positive thing; that they were a good indicator that I was ovulating both regularly and normally. And so I thought that the first step of my fertility investigations was going to be pretty straightforward. I thought that I didn't have too much to worry about, that the test to make sure that I was ovulating normally would be just a formality. And I suppose that goes to show just how very wrong you can be.

We received the results of my blood test in the post. We skimmed them, we studied them, we pored over them, we looked up the most incomprehensible bits on the Internet and in our dictionary but we still didn't really understand them. I have always had a deeply ingrained sense of fear of any news that is delivered with seemingly deliberate incomprehensibility. In my years of working in marketing, I had learnt how to dress up bad news with jargon to conceal the worst of it, to soften the blow, and I was beginning to suspect that the medical profession wasn't any different. I needed to get some straight answers. And so I phoned the health centre and, with just the tiniest of hints at the rising panic that I was finding increasingly difficult to control, I managed to secure a between-appointments slot for Paul and me, for an informal chat with the nurse. It was something that I seemed to be getting incredibly good at, conjuring up health centre appointments out of thin air.

Paul and I wasted no time in explaining our situation. We told the nurse that we had been trying for a baby, without success, for over two years. We told her that Paul had already been checked out and that his sperm count was fine. And we told her that the results from my initial blood test had come back and that we were mortified because they seemed to suggest that I wasn't ovulating. The nurse was instantly sympathetic toward us and, attempting to allay our fears, she opened up my file on her PC. She told us that she would explain the blood test's findings to both of us, in layman's terms.

My medical notes appeared on the computer screen and I scanned over the words at an impressively breakneck speed. Admittedly, my impressive speed was largely due to the fact that I was skipping over the bits that I didn't understand (about 95 per cent of them). And then my eyes alighted on the phrase, 'suggests premature menopause' and as my brain registered the significance of those three little words, my speed-reading ground to a halt, my heart missed several beats and total numbness took hold of my body. I was frozen. And my eyes were locked, unblinkingly, onto the computer screen in front of me until the nurse broke into my stunned silence when she had eventually read on to the same place in my notes.

'Now, stop whatever it is that you are thinking. Please. This could mean absolutely anything.' The nurse did her best to reassure us, 'Maybe you were stressed out about the blood test, Isla. Maybe it was just one of those months when ovulation didn't happen – it's not uncommon ... In fact the blood test might even have been done on the wrong day. The timing of these things has to be spot on, you know.'

The nurse registered the stricken expression on both of our faces. 'Look, I'll ask the doctor to squeeze you in at the end of surgery. She'll be able to explain it all to you. She'll make a better job of it than me.'

Paul and I stumbled blindly through the waiting room and out into the car park, the words 'premature menopause' hanging heavily and ominously between us. And we waited for surgery to end.

Bringing in the Specialists

My doctor seemed to have two very distinct approaches to appointments with her patients.

The first: '*You* are a moron – you know effectively nothing and, consequently, *I* am going to use words of two syllables or less.'

The second: '*You* seem as though you are an intelligent person and so you will instantly understand complex biological theories that took me several years at medical school to acquire.'

Flattering though it was to receive a consultation in the latter style, nothing that my doctor could say – and certainly not the bits that I understood – could reassure me in any way. And her eventual suggestion that we were referred to a specialist – to a consultant specializing in the treatment of *infertility* – was absolutely the last thing that I needed to hear. For me, this referral to a fertility specialist seemed to bring little hope that this problem of ours was something that could be resolved quickly and easily to a rather abrupt end.

Shell-shocked, Paul and I made our way out and the nurse collared us in the waiting room. She didn't wait for a response to her question, 'How did it go?' I think the stunned expression on both of our faces told her everything that she needed to know.

'Look, don't worry. I've got a feeling that I'm going to be seeing the pair of you at antenatal classes before the year is out.'

And although the nurse couldn't possibly have known what was around the corner for us, someone else's optimism gave my own the tiniest of boosts.

Surfing for Answers

Unfortunately my company's medical insurance scheme didn't run to fertility specialists and, even if it had, I don't think that I would have felt comfortable sharing that particular information with my workmates. Paranoid, I could imagine the round-the-photocopier conversations. 'Hey, you'll never guess who can't have kids ...'

But without the benefit of queue jumping, my appointment with the fertility specialist seemed to be a long time coming. So, in the meantime, I began to lose myself for hours, surfing the Internet at work. Looking for clues, looking for answers, looking for solutions. Looking for a glimmer of hope to cling to. Looking for something, looking for *anything*. And although I limited myself, at first, to lunchtime surfing when the office was more likely to be quiet, I quickly found myself sneaking in fertility-related Internet searches at every possible opportunity. I lost track of the amount of times that I desperately had to minimize my PC's screen as yet another uninvited visitor popped their head around my office door. I was keenly aware that I would be hard pushed to explain away highly technical, biological drawings of the female reproductive system as work-related.

When I was a kid, I developed an unhealthy fascination with the family medical encyclopaedia. I would pore over the book for hours on end absorbing the gory details of a myriad of diseases. Despite knowing rationally, even at the time, that a strangulated testicle was highly unlikely – OK, a physical impossibility for a pre-pubescent girl – I would still be able to convince myself that I was exhibiting the symptoms of a textbook example of the condition. Some twenty years later and my net-surfing on fertility-impacting complaints began to have much the same result.

I quickly became convinced that I was suffering from every single infertility-causing ailment that I happened to click upon. I became convinced that I was suffering from PCOS and from fibroids, from chlamydia and from anaemia, from endometriosis and from a defective luteal phase. I became convinced that I was suffering from both a progesterone deficiency and from an oestrogen deficiency – despite the two conditions being, generally, mutually exclusive. I became convinced that I was overweight and that I was underweight. That I was too stressed out and chilled out. And I became convinced that I was too old.

Website after website cheerily informed me that women possess their optimum baby making powers while they are still in their teens. After that, it was pretty much downhill all the way to thirty-five, by which time women had effectively had it. So that was it. Time was running out for me. I had started trying for a baby too damned late. And, time travel aside, there was absolutely nothing that I could do about it.

'We're Going in ...'

Several weeks after an initial and surprisingly brief consultation with the fertility specialist up at our local hospital, my appointment date arrived for the recommended next step in my fertility investigations. An appointment for something called a laparoscopy, something that I had discovered was an investigative (and invasive) procedure. I had supplemented the sketchy details that I had received about the procedure from the fertility specialist with (surprise, surprise) my own Internet research findings. And so I felt as though I had a pretty good idea of what to expect.

I knew that I was going to need to have a general anaesthetic, for a start. And I knew that a tiny incision was going to have to be made near my belly button so that a minute camera could be inserted, to get a closer look at my internal reproductive system. I knew that a second incision would have to be made too, an inch or so further down from the first one, to allow gas to be introduced, to distend my entire pelvic area and to give the fertility specialist a much clearer picture of just what exactly was going on in there. I knew that dye was going to be injected into my fallopian tubes to ensure that they were blockage-free. And consequently, I would have a blue vaginal discharge for a day or two afterwards. And that, although it was going to be

'We're Going in ...'   41

peculiar in appearance, a blue vaginal discharge, in this particular instance, was no cause for alarm; in fact a blue vaginal discharge was actually a good thing, because it meant that the injected dye had been able to pass freely through my tubes.

I also knew that after the operation my shoulders were likely to be uncomfortable for a bit, as any last remnant of gas rose up through my body, trying its hardest to escape. I knew that I was going to feel groggy for a few days afterwards, because of the anaesthetic and because of the shock to the system, of an operation. I knew that I would need to take a couple of days off work and that I would need to rest, to let my body recover. In other words, I knew that my laparoscopy was going to be a piece of cake.

My period was due on the day of my laparoscopy, so I also knew that I was going to need to have a pregnancy test before the fertility specialist could go ahead with the procedure – poking about with cameras, gas and dye presumably not being particularly conducive to any early pregnancy proceeding safely and healthily to full term. God, I had imagined that scenario over and over again in my head – the nurse going off with the blood sample for my pregnancy test and then coming back into the consulting room with a grin that she could barely suppress.

'Well, Mrs McGuckin, judging by the result of your pregnancy test, it looks as though the operation isn't going to be necessary after all …'

No such luck. An hour later, the pregnancy test result had come back negative and I was being wheeled into theatre.

'How Long Have I got, Doctor?'

I don't know what exactly Paul had been expecting to see when he arrived to collect me from the hospital later that day. Maybe he thought that I would be up and about already. Maybe he thought that I would be still in bed, but that I would be cheery and chirpy and chatting to the other patients on the ward. But the reality of the sight of me, looking faintly green and just barely upright, propped up with pillows in my hospital bed, was obviously way too much for him. Within half an hour of him arriving on the ward, the nurses had Paul installed in a comfy arm chair close to an open window and were giving him sips of iced water to quell his dizziness. There was even some debate – and only half of it was banter – about which one of us was going to be the safest to drive home.

The pair of us managed to recover our faculties a bit. And by the time that the fertility specialist had begun his rounds of the ward, Paul and I were as *compos mentis* as we were ever going to be. I had known before the operation that the fertility specialist would be able to let us know pretty much straightaway what, if anything, the laparoscopy had uncovered. And so, of course, I had developed various scenarios in my head.

Everything from: 'Well, Mrs McGuckin, we did find a tiny little blockage in one of your fallopian tubes but, with a gentle gust of air, we have managed to completely clear it. Everything will be OK now and I can personally guarantee that you will be pregnant before the month is out.'

To: 'I'm terribly sorry, Mrs McGuckin, but you are missing most of the basic biological equipment required in order to conceive. It would be a medical impossibility for you ever to become pregnant.'

And to be honest, even the latter scenario would have been preferable to the reality; that the cause of our infertility continued to be unexplained. The fertility specialist wasted no time in breaking the rather disappointing news to us.

'We didn't find anything. Your fallopian tubes are clear and everything else seems to be functioning perfectly normally. And although you do have a touch of endometriosis, it really is very common, nothing at all to worry about and certainly nothing that would affect your fertility.'

What a bloody anti-climax. In a surprising show of sensitivity, the fertility specialist picked up on my obvious frustration.

'Lots of women find that the operation itself has a sort of spring cleaning effect and that they get pregnant very soon afterwards. Fingers crossed, eh?'

Yes, fingers crossed.

Sex 'n' Drugs 'n' Hot Flushes

It seemed that my finger-crossing technique was proving to be as woefully inadequate as my leg uncrossing one. It seemed that I wasn't going to be one of the women who were lucky enough to get pregnant as soon as they had come round from the laparoscopy's anaesthetic. Three months later, Paul and I were in the fertility specialist's consulting room once more, discussing fertility drugs and their seemingly never-ending list of side effects. Some sensitive soul (not) had already cheerfully informed me that Clomid – the ovulation-enhancing drug of my fertility specialist's choice – was carcinogenic. And so the pessimist in me had muttered, 'Bloody typical, knowing your luck you'll end up with cancer instead of a baby.'

Still, I tried hard to focus on the more typical side effects that the fertility specialist was describing to us. Side effects like hot flushes and nausea, blurred vision and mood swings. And, despite all of them sounding horrendous, I was prepared to endure whatever side effects Clomid threw at me if the fertility drug was going to help me to conceive.

'What's next?' Paul had asked, as the fertility specialist handed me a prescription for a three-month course of the drugs, 'If Clomid doesn't work?'

'Well, we'll have a go at IUI first and then we'll move on to IVF.' Just like that.

I was incredulous. I couldn't believe how matter-of-fact the fertility specialist was managing to be about the painful reality of our situation. It was as though the seriousness of it all, the almost unbearable sadness of it all, had somehow just passed him by. Paul and I weren't going to be able to make a baby – we weren't going to be able to do what other happy and loving couples do – without medical intervention. And all of a sudden, and almost without realizing it, it seemed as though we were on some kind of hideous roller coaster.

And I was terrified. Terrified by the prospect of invasive medical procedures that had been described to me in cold and clinical language that I only half understood. But as terrified as I was, I really didn't feel as though getting off that fertility treatment roller coaster – taking the opportunity to catch my breath, collect my thoughts and consider the alternatives – was an option for me. I was as terrified about getting *off* the roller coaster as I was about staying on it. I was terrified about getting off the roller coaster in case there was a baby waiting for Paul and me at the end of it. And because I was feeling frightened and frustrated and, let's face it, because I was feeling incredibly sorry for myself and despite the expression of absolute horror on the fertility specialist's face, I burst into tears.

Life's Not Fair

We handed over the prescription for my fertility drugs and we waited our turn at the hospital pharmacy. I was still sobbing, loudly and snottily, and other people in the waiting room were beginning to stare at me, presumably making the assumption that I had just been diagnosed with something terminal. And I really did feel as though I had been.

Everywhere I looked, there were people with kids. There were loads of people with sick kids, too. And I know that that was not entirely unreasonable in a hospital pharmacy waiting room, but I couldn't help thinking that if the parents of those kids had had to try as hard as Paul and I were doing in order to conceive, they would have taken better care of their kids, they wouldn't have been so negligent as parents that they let their kids get sick. Eventually I managed to avert my gaze from the crèche for sick children that was forming in front of us and let my eyes wander beyond the waiting room and outside, to a couple of smokers huddled together, companionably. When my gaze drifted closer to ground level, I spotted the children with them, and had to almost physically restrain myself from running outside and snatching their children away from them, from shrieking at them, 'Don't make them breathe your smoke, you selfish, selfish bastards!'

Not a moment too soon, the prescription for my fertility drugs was ready and Paul and I could return to the sanctuary of our car. My tears had continued pretty much unabated since leaving the fertility specialist's office and they became even more angry and more bitter as we sat in the car park. Valiantly, Paul attempted to console me – a thankless and impossible task – before he would even consider driving away. What seemed like just a matter of seconds after we had got into our car, would-be parkers began to circle us in theirs. Like sharks. They wordlessly gestured to us, 'You going?' And I knew that it was highly unlikely that they were searching for a hospital car parking space for fun. I knew that they were probably experiencing an equally – if not even more – difficult time of their own. And yet still I couldn't stop myself from angrily, but equally wordlessly, gesturing right back at them.

The Drugs ...

On day one of my next cycle – or the first day of my next period in less medical speak – I made the decision to go ahead and give my reproductive system the kick up the backside that it so obviously needed. So, with no small amount of trepidation, I took my first Clomid tablet. Paul had an almost superstitious feeling that if those fertility drugs were going to work for us at all, they would work on the first attempt. And, because a friend of a friend (there always seemed to be someone, somewhere) had struggled to get pregnant for years but had then managed to conceive on *her* first Clomid cycle, I felt as though the clock had started ticking for me, the second that I swallowed that very first tablet. The stakes were high and the pressure was on and all that we could do was wait and hope.

I knew, deep down, that the likelihood was for *any* fertility treatment to fail rather than to succeed. And I knew that fertility drugs like Clomid were only ever a first step, a maybe, just a maybe. But none of that could have stopped my hopes from being raised when I was ever so slightly sick one morning, a few days before my period was due. (Sick, for God's sake, and in the morning!!!) But my hopes became gradually, and then totally, dashed as my usual pre-menstrual madness began. I cleaned the house from top to bottom. I tidied the cutlery drawer, rearranging the spoons, the forks, and the knives. And then I noticed it. The spot on my chin – same place, same time, every month. You could set your clock based on the day and time that spot appeared. I cried at an *Eastenders'* storyline. I cried at a song on the radio. I cried at a particularly heart-warming TV ad. And I started an absolutely horrendous period on the day of my work Christmas party. And then I cried some more. Merry bloody Christmas.

... Don't Work

Of course it is easy to say all of this, looking back and with the perfect clarity – the 20:20 vision – of hindsight, but I did have my doubts about Clomid from the start. I had my doubts about what exactly the drug could do for me. Despite my anxiety-inducing episode with ovulation testing at my local health centre, I was fairly sure that I was ovulating normally. I had a feeling that the nurse down at the health centre had been right, that it was just the timing of the test that had been wrong. My gynaecologist had told me that my painful and regular periods were a pretty good indicator of a functional ovulatory cycle – that I was probably releasing an egg, in other words. And, of course, my frequent searches on the Internet had provided me with plenty of other ovulation occurrence clues to look out for:

'Mittelschmerz' or middle pain – Slight twinge, mid-cycle, uncomfortable rather than painful, usually on the right hand side.

Check. Every month without fail.

EWCM or egg white cervical mucus – Highly distinctive in its clarity, in its stretchability and in its slipperiness

Check. Ditto.

And so the logic of being prescribed a course of fertility drugs just seems to escape me. If I was ovulating as normally and as regularly as I appeared to be and if the whole point of fertility drugs like Clomid was to correct ovulation irregularities, then what was the point of me taking it? Looking back, goodness only knows why I didn't just ask my fertility specialist that very question.

It was as though my inability to conceive had taken away my self-confidence, too. It was difficult, impossible even, to believe in myself as a strong and intelligent woman. If I wasn't going to be able to have children, then I felt as though I was a pretty poor excuse for a woman. Never mind a strong woman, or an intelligent one. And so I remember feeling incredibly powerless. And I remember feeling confused, as though I was trapped in some sort of vague and fuzzy bubble. I think I might have been in a state of shock, actually. I certainly couldn't get my head around the label of infertility – unexplained or otherwise – that had been applied to Paul and myself. I couldn't get my head around the necessity of consultations with a fertility specialist, either, or the necessity of fertility treatment.

And because I felt confused, because I felt *powerless*, I think that I just handed over the responsibility for my fertility. I just gave up. I started to believe that my own body didn't know what it needed to do in order to get pregnant. I started to believe that my own body just didn't have a clue. And I needed to believe that the fertility specialist *did* have a clue. That the fertility specialist knew best, about what was best for my body, about what was best for me. That he knew the best course of action to take in order to help me to get pregnant. And so I didn't really feel as though I should question him about the appropriateness of fertility drugs for me. So I kept quiet. I did what I was told to do. I persevered and took the drug for four consecutive cycles. Knowing that when the fourth cycle of drugs didn't work – I had quickly reached the stage where I could no longer muster a positive outlook, where I could no longer say 'if the fourth cycle of drugs didn't work', not even to myself – I was going to be faced with Intra Uterine Insemination. IUI. And then the fury kicked in.

Personality Transplant

I had been warned that fertility drugs could cause mood swings; that they could have quite marked emotional side effects; I had even heard of Clomid being described as 'Hormone Hell', but I was still quite unprepared for the effect that fertility drugs had on me – and Paul, and on any other poor soul who had the misfortune of incurring my wrath.

'How dare they? HOW DARE THEY?'

Paul had learned from bitter experience that there could be no correct answer to this question and so he kept his mouth firmly shut as I hurled my magazine across the room. And the catalyst for this particular outburst? I had wanted our baby's name to be original. I had wanted it to be unique. Not just some kind of sad me-too, copied from a C-list celebrity, the arrival of whose baby seemed to be plastered across every single magazine that I happened to open. I was furious. Again. And I carefully selected another imagined slight from my well-stocked arsenal – a conversation with a friend that had really infuriated me. And I let rip.

'And can you believe that she actually sat there and told me that she wasn't going to ask me any more, about how the fertility treatment was going? How selfish is that? How hurtful? Well, I'm sorry that it's all got so very boring – hearing about my continued inability to conceive. But I thought that's what friends were for. Being there and supporting you through the good times and the bad.' I came up for breath before delivering my killer line, 'and I like to think that if I had had cancer the novelty of talking to me about *that* wouldn't have worn off quite so damn quickly.'

Although he was canny enough not to contradict me during these tirades, Paul knew that that wasn't what my friend had meant. And, not so very deep down, so did I. My friend didn't want to keep asking me about my fertility treatment because she didn't want me to feel as though she was badgering me. She didn't want me to feel as though she was nagging me. That she was putting even more pressure on me when I was already quite clearly getting dangerously close to breaking point. But I didn't want to see things that way. It suited my frame of my mind to believe that the world and his dog were out to get me.

A Problem Shared

‘I think I’m going round the bloody twist, slowly but ever so surely.’ After Sunday lunch and a few glasses of wine round at my brother’s house, I was in a reflective mood.

‘I fly off the handle about the slightest little thing these days. And the big things – like just about all of my friends announcing their pregnancies month after month after month – well, I just can’t cope with them. I know that I can’t expect my friends to put their baby making plans on hold just because I don’t seem to be able to get pregnant. And I know that they don’t really expect me to be jumping for joy when I hear yet more “happy” news. But it just feels as though no one can do or say the right thing at the minute. Not any of my newly pregnant friends and certainly not me. If my friends come straight out with it – “I’m pregnant!” – I’m offended by their bluntness, by their lack of tact. And I rehearse, over and over in my head, the perfectly tactful and emotionally intelligent way that I would convey such news to someone who had been trying for a baby for over two years. But, then again, if my friends try and break their news to me gently, I’m furious, incensed by their pity. And then I feel guilty ...’

‘Guilty?’

'Yeah. About turning into such an evil bitch that I can't honestly be happy for my own friends any more. And, of course, I would be absolutely mortified to think that any one of them could pick up on even the tiniest hint of the anger and the jealousy and the bitterness that I've got simmering away inside.'

'Have you thought about going to see someone?'

'Like who?' Dear Lord, I remember thinking, if my sister-in-law was seriously going to suggest that I needed to see a shrink, things must have been even worse than I had thought.

'Like a homeopath.'

Like a Homeopath

I didn't know much about homeopathy. In fact I didn't really know anything about homeopathy. I would have been happy to have spent my first appointment just getting to know what homeopathy involved and what it could cure and – let's be honest, here – what it could do for me, what it could do to improve my chances of having a baby. Although the homeopath obligingly filled in the considerable gaps in my knowledge about homeopathy ...

That it has been around for hundreds of years.

That it is based on the principle that like can cure like. Despite caffeine not being renowned as being especially conducive to a good night's sleep, for example, it is believed that a minute dose of coffee can help to cure insomnia.

That it recognizes symptoms of ill health as expressions of disharmony within the whole person; so it treats the patient not just the disease, stimulating the body's own defences and immune processes to help the body to heal itself.

... the real benefit of that first appointment was the opportunity to just talk to someone. I knew almost instinctively and before my homeopath had described to me her professional code of conduct and client confidentiality that I could say to her whatever I liked. That I could let the words just come tumbling out. Knowing that whatever I said would go no further. That whatever I said would be heard without somebody else jumping in with their own experiences, with their own advice; that whatever I said would be heard without judgement. That I could talk about my hopes – about having a baby, about having a family, about shaking off that millstone of infertility. And about my fears that I was rapidly turning into one of those women who I used to pity; one of those women who have become so desperate for a baby that they no longer care about the cost to themselves or to their partner or to their relationship. I could talk to my homeopath about my feelings about all of those things, too. About my growing sense of futility and of sadness, my growing sense of anger and of frustration.

I relayed a conversation to my homeopath; one that I had had with a friend who had asked me if I had considered adoption. Without skipping a beat, I had replied, 'Yes, but not as often as I've considered suicide.' And I had been shocked to realize, at the time, that I was only half joking.

And I told my homeopath about my thoughts on IVF. I just went through the motions, at first, listing all of the logical and rational reasons why I had decided not to try it. Not just yet.

'It would just feel too invasive somehow, as though I was tampering with nature. And I'm really worried about the effect that it would have on our relationship, about the strain that it would put us both under. The pressure.'

And then I paused before blurting out something that I hadn't even allowed myself to think before. 'I'm terrified, too. Because if IVF doesn't work, that's it, isn't it? It's the end of the road for us. There's nothing else left to try.'

And then the homeopath asked me about my diet and my periods, my sleeping patterns and my stress levels. And I asked her why she thought that I hadn't conceived yet. In addition to the goodness knows how many years that she had spent studying homeopathic remedies, it was clear that my homeopath had also acquired some rock-solid counselling skills somewhere along the way. She threw my question straight back at me.

'Why do *you* think that you haven't conceived yet?'

My reply was out of my mouth before my brain had even fully registered the question, 'I think that we've just been spectacularly unlucky.' And I hoped that, one day soon, our luck was going to change.

TomCat?!

I didn't realize, at the time, just how significant it was – my first appointment with a homeopath, my first appointment with any sort of alternative practitioner. Looking back, that appointment was the first, rather tentative step on my journey toward embracing a much more natural, much more holistic way of living. And, like so many of life's most important journeys, for me that journey has often been a case of one step forward and two steps back.

I would really love to be able to say that I got pregnant that month, the month after I had my first appointment with the homeopath and I had taken my first homeopathic remedy. But it wouldn't be true. Paul and I were far too busy climbing on to the next rung of the fertility treatment ladder – for Intra Uterine Insemination. For IUI.

The IUI experience really does seem to vary dramatically. It seems to depend on things like the procedural preferences of the fertility specialist involved, and even on details like postcodes, because postcodes determine the catchment area for any particular fertility clinic. I had a friend who lived in a different part of town and attended a different fertility clinic to me. My friend got lucky and she was offered the all-singing, all-dancing version of IUI. And my friend got pregnant.

The very first time that she tried it. I have a sneaking suspicion that I was offered the bargain basement version of IUI.

Whatever the version, the man's bit of the IUI process is basically the same. He is provided with a sterile container and he is expected to do the five-knuckle-shuffle into it – not an easy task, I am told – without spilling half of the container's contents. He then has to rush the filled container along to a laboratory at the fertility clinic so that its contents can be washed and spun, ready for the next stage. And, ideally, he has to do that within half an hour of ejaculation. And that was where things got slightly tricky for Paul. At the time, Paul and I lived at least forty-five minutes away from the hospital where our fertility clinic was situated. And that was on a good day – with no rush hour traffic to contend with and no unexpected hold-ups and no road works. So Paul was left with three choices, each excruciatingly unappealing in their own different way:

Option 1: Grab a furtive five minutes with a well-thumbed magazine in a cold, lonely and sterile cubicle at the hospital.

Option 2: Take up the offer of a bathroom from a close-to-the-hospital friend. Trying not to be too distracted from the job in hand by the repetitive strains of the Tweenies' theme tune, as our friend used the rare treat of non-stop DVDs in an attempt to take her toddlers' minds off the fact that Uncle Paul had been in the bathroom for a very long time.

Option 3: Do the business in his office loo.

Decisions, decisions, eh? After some deliberation, Paul eventually chose the latter of the three evils and locked himself away in his office loo with an appropriately stimulating magazine. He managed to ignore shouts from a colleague such as, 'Fancy a cuppa Paul?' as she passed the firmly locked toilet door on the way to the kitchen. He tried not to feel too vulnerable as he passed the same colleague on his way out trying valiantly to keep the little pot and its contents upright in his trouser pocket. Then he made his excuses, 'I'm just heading out for an hour' and left, to meet me up at the hospital, at the fertility clinic.

Whether it is the all-singing, all-dancing version or the bargain basement one, IUI is a fairly low-tech procedure and a pretty quick one, too. Very much, 'Wham bam, thank you, ma'am'. All that I had to do was to take off my tights and knickers, lie down on an examination table and get the best of Paul's bunch injected into me using a very thin and very flexible catheter. A 'Tomcat' catheter, no less. The whole experience did start to get a bit surreal when the nurse brought a cup of tea for us both afterwards. I did half expect her to come back with a post-coital cigarette for us, too. But she didn't. And that was that. My first IUI treatment. Done and dusted.

The Bargain Basement of NHS Fertility Treatment ...?

IUI can work, of course it can. And it does work, for some lucky couples. It had worked for my friend, for my friend with the luckier postcode. And so I wanted to know what the chances were of it working for us. I wanted to know if Paul and I were going to get lucky, too. So I got busy with my favourite websites and I did a bit of research into the subject.

I discovered that IUI was far more likely to work for couples where sperm count was an issue or for couples where there was a problem with the quality or the quantity of cervical mucus – I read that, in some extreme cases, cervical mucus could create hostile or even impenetrable conditions for sperm. And, according to my research, I found out that the most important function of IUI treatment, its real *raison d'être*, was in getting sperm to the right place – like as close to where the egg is released as possible – and at the right time. And so, I discovered, it was usually helpful during IUI treatment to make sure that there was an egg around when the sperm was injected in.

Apparently, human eggs are only viable for a maximum of twenty-four hours after they have been released, so with IUI timing really is everything. In an ideal world, IUI treatment would be carried out within six hours before or after ovulation – no matter what time of the day or night that turned out to be. Some fertility clinics advocate the use of a whole host of ovulation detection techniques to make sure that the timing of the IUI treatment is as close to perfect as it can be. Some clinics use basal body temperature and urine tests to detect the hormonal surges that indicate that ovulation is about to take place. Some use a combination of fertility drugs and blood tests to determine optimum timing. Some monitor follicular development using ultrasound scans.

But that wasn't the case with my fertility clinic. I was advised to just carry on taking my Clomid tablets while the timing of my IUI treatments was based on the first day of my last period. Give or take a few days if the perfect moment happened to fall during out-of-clinic hours, or over the weekend. Or on a Bank Holiday Monday. Hmm. It certainly didn't seem to me to be the most scientific of approaches – not when the timing of IUI treatment was so very crucial. But Paul and I had read that optimism was one of the most important things when you are trying to conceive, when you are undergoing fertility treatment. And so, optimistic we tried to stay.

Off-Games Week (and Other Euphemisms)

When you have made the decision to start trying for a baby, there is something about the onset of a period that seems particularly unfair. I felt as though each period was a painful, bloody and emotionally disruptive reminder that our attempts to have a baby had been unsuccessful. And somehow that sense of unfairness was made even worse – like about a hundred times worse – because Paul and I had had to resort to invasive fertility treatment in our quest to conceive. The pressure seemed to mount with each month that passed and with every unsuccessful cycle of fertility treatment. I felt all too aware that the number of treatment options available to us was dwindling rapidly. My periods seemed to come around more quickly with every month that passed. And with every month that passed I felt painfully aware of time marching, relentlessly, on.

I found it really hard to strike the right emotional balance. Some months I would be ludicrously optimistic, pre-menstrually. I would raise my hopes up to the rafters and pounce gleefully on the slightest little physical symptom – anything that could (oh please, God, please) indicate an early pregnancy. Symptoms like an inexplicable twinge in my side. Like painfully swollen breasts or an unusual and metallic taste in my mouth.

Like a fleeting sensation of sickness or of dizziness. And I would read deep and meaningful significance into the most obscure of 'signs'. Signs like a sudden and nausea-invoking aversion to coffee, for example. Or like the uncharacteristic friendliness of my usually aloof – and, frankly, cat-like – cat. I would convince myself that the cat knew something that I didn't, that cats had some sort of innate sixth sense about that type of thing, that she was attempting to secure her place in my affections before a tiny human usurper came along.

And then some months I would swing to the other extreme. I would talk myself into 'knowing' that the fertility treatment hadn't been a success. I would tell myself that I didn't need my period to start to know that I wasn't pregnant. And then I would tell myself that I wasn't particularly bothered anyway, about having a baby. It was an attempt at some kind of reverse psychology I suppose, trying to tempt fate – beware of what you *don't* wish for …

But no matter what mind games I tried to play with myself on those downbeat months, I couldn't quite shake off a growing sense of failure. A feeling that seemed to become heightened with every month that passed, with every missed opportunity. As the months passed, I began to see each period as a literally painful reminder that, yet again, my baby wish – and what had started to feel as though it was my *only* wish had not been granted.

And yet, despite the reality of extremely low success rates with IUI – according to some sources, success rates that were as low as single figure percentages, even for the all-singing, all-dancing versions of the treatment – and despite my research telling me that the treatment was far from tailor made to my and Paul's particular needs, after my first attempt at IUI, my emotional pendulum swung firmly toward the ludicrously optimistic. I even did a pregnancy test – I had managed to get myself so totally and utterly convinced that my fertility treatment had been successful. It was a nail biting few minutes' wait until I saw the little blue line which meant that the pregnancy test had worked, and just a second or two more before I registered the absence of a second little blue line which meant that the IUI treatment hadn't. But so very ludicrous was my sense of optimism that month that for a few happily deluded hours I almost talked myself into believing that I was the 0.001 percent in the 99.999 percent pregnancy test effectiveness ratio. I almost talked myself into believing that the test was wrong, that I *was* pregnant. But it wasn't, and I wasn't, and my period started later on that day.

I once read a rather poetic description of menstrual blood being tears of sadness from the womb. Tears that the womb was crying for a much longed-for baby. Tears that the womb was crying for a baby that she so desperately wanted to hold and to protect and to nurture. And, after my first failed attempt at IUI, I could empathize completely with how my disappointed womb must have been feeling. Because I can remember a feeling of complete and utter desolation as I picked up the phone to tell my closest friends and family the unhappy news that once again Paul and I were losers in the fertility treatment lottery.

Third Time Lucky?

The months passed and the day arrived for yet another appointment up at the fertility clinic, an appointment for my third attempt out of a recommended series of four IUI treatments. Paul had taken his special delivery up to the fertility clinic earlier that morning but then he had to head off somewhere, off to a work related meeting of some sort, something that he really couldn't get out of. So, after he had done his bit, I had to go through the rest of that third IUI procedure alone.

I don't think that I had ever really understood what being alone felt like until that day. I had certainly never felt quite so small or so vulnerable as I did lying there on that examination couch after my third IUI treatment, my bare legs bent at the knee in an attempt to let gravity give the just-injected semen as fighting a chance as possible. And for a while, as I lay there, I just let myself wallow – rather indulgently I think, looking back, rather theatrically – in a wave of desolation and of sadness, of self pity and of loneliness. And then I started to cry and I let myself acknowledge just how desperately unhappy I had become about our situation. I let myself cry because I felt frustrated and I felt sad about our continued inability to conceive. I let myself cry because of the indignity and the seeming futility of the fertility treatment that Paul and I were undergoing. I let myself cry because it all just seemed so very unfair. And then I tried to stop myself from crying. I tried to pull myself together. Aware that I needed to get myself up and get myself dressed, that I needed to free up the room for the next unfortunate fertility patient.

And I was surprised to find that I couldn't stop crying. Not at first. Not until my tears had eventually dissolved into a very real sense of anger. And God was I angry. I was angry about our unexplained infertility, our involuntary childlessness. I was angry about being there in that fertility clinic, alone. I was angry about what seemed like coldness – what seemed like indifference – from the fertility specialist. But most of all I was angry – I was furious – that I had allowed myself to be railroaded into such an emotionally and physically punishing regime of fertility treatment that, at the end of the day, seemed far from tailor made to our particular needs.

If I was ovulating normally and I was fairly sure that I was why had I been prescribed a course of fertility drugs that were supposed to stimulate ovulation? And I had already taken seven lots of Clomid without success. I had put on weight. I had developed spots. I had suffered from hot flushes and mood swings. It seemed as though the only side effect that I hadn't managed to succumb to was pregnancy.

And if Paul's sperm count really was as hunky dory as his test results had indicated, why was I being subjected to Intra Uterine Insemination? When IUI was an invasive and in my experience a highly stressful fertility treatment that only seemed to offer any real hope for couples where low sperm count was an issue?

And if the holy grail of successful IUI treatment was timing, then why was I being treated on Wednesday lunchtime when I was pretty damn sure – and I had told my fertility specialist as much – that I had ovulated the Monday before?

And I started to worry, too. What if I *had* already conceived, earlier that week, naturally? Would the IUI treatment itself, not to mention all of the stress and all of the frustration and all of the anxiety that surrounded the procedure for me, have jeopardized that potential conception in some way? And, as I pulled on my socks and shoes, I can remember thinking, 'I just wish that this was all over, so that I could concentrate on getting pregnant ...'

Time Out

After our third attempt at IUI we had a very long chat, Paul and me, a real heart to heart.

'It was just so *desperate* today – even more desperate than usual. I suppose part of it was because you weren't there but … Oh, I don't know. I just thought that fertility treatment was supposed to give you *hope*.'

'I know exactly what you mean. I don't think I've ever felt *less* hopeful about our chances of having a baby than when the specialist prescribed those fertility drugs for you. I hated hearing about all of those side effects, hated what you were going to have to go through.'

'I know. And it's funny. Now that we're seeing a specialist and having fertility treatment – I feel as though we are infertile.'

'Yeah. What's the word for it? A self-fulfilling prophecy. We're seeing a fertility specialist, so we *must* be infertile. Even though it's unexplained, our infertility, it still *is* infertility. Isn't it?'

'Yeah and what a depressing, hopeless kind of word that is. Infertility. It makes me feel as though the pair of us are completely beyond hope when it comes to having babies. It makes me feel as though our chances of ever having a baby – never mind an entire *family* – are slim to non-existent.'

It *was* a difficult decision to make, looking back; I am still pretty sure that it was the right one. Both Paul and I felt in urgent need of some time out and so we made the decision not to go ahead with our fourth attempt at IUI. We made the decision to have a complete break from fertility treatment for a year or so, to just let nature take its course, to wait and see what the next twelve months would bring us. And, once we had made up our minds, the sense of relief – for both of us – was almost indescribable. No more trips to the fertility clinic. No more drugs. No more IUI. We could start to make love again instead of making do with 'trying-for-a-baby sex' because our calendar told us that we had to. And, strangely, I started to feel more positive than I had done in a long time, about a family-filled future for us. Part of me was convinced that now we had put a stop to the whole palaver of trying for a baby, to the whole time-consuming business of fertility treatment, I was going to find myself pregnant. One day, very soon.

You Are What You Eat (So I Must Have Been a Microwaveable Ready Meal)

I put my previously all-encompassing goal of getting pregnant firmly on to the back burner for a while. My new goal was to get myself into the pink of health – mind, body and soul. I decided to tackle my diet first. I had always loved food. And, where finances, time and the availability of decent ingredients had allowed, I would usually choose a fairly healthy and well-balanced diet for myself; one with lots of fruit and vegetables, one with lots of salads and fresh fish, one with lots of brown rice and wholemeal bread. All of the good stuff, all of the *nutritious* stuff.

But the busier I had got at work, the more heavily I had started to rely on convenience food. I started to buy ready meals because they were tasty enough, because they were readily available – our local twenty-four hour petrol station had a mind-boggling selection – and, let's face it, I bought them because they were quick. And so they were an increasingly tempting option after the hour or more in rush hour traffic that, for me, concluded an everyday working day that had started creeping ever closer to twelve hours.

I suppose I knew deep down, though, that there had to be a pay off. I knew that there was no such thing as a free lunch – proverbial or otherwise. And I decided to stop burying my head in the sand, to wake up to the facts about processed food. I didn't need to read the scare stories that appeared in the weekend newspapers – week after week after week – common sense told me everything that I needed to know. That during the manufacturing process, for example, refined foods can be stripped, sometimes almost entirely, of their original nutrients. That the longer shelf lives that made these food products 'oh-so-convenient' for people like me could have a profoundly detrimental effect on their food values. That the freshest and the juiciest looking of fruit and vegetables could well have lost most of their vitamin and mineral content in transit; that their appealing appearance on the supermarket shelf may have had more to do with preservatives and pesticides than with nutritional value. That even fresh meat could contain traces of growth hormones – great news, presumably, for the profit levels of the meat producers who could turn calves into cows almost overnight, but not such great news for those couples who were struggling to conceive, who really didn't need to be ingesting anything that was going to affect the balance of their hormone levels, however minutely.

I started to pore over labels and ingredients in the supermarket. If there was an ingredient that I couldn't pronounce or one that I wouldn't recognize if I saw it on a plate, the product wouldn't make it as far as my shopping basket. I cut out as much processed stuff as I could without becoming neurotic. I chose organic food wherever possible. And I also decided to do something about my caffeine and alcohol intake.

The Future is DeCaf (and Alcohol-free)

It is funny, how the moment you start to become aware of something, you notice it everywhere. I seemed to read newspaper article after newspaper article informing me about the toxicity of the world, telling me about how our entire planet is awash with fertility-zapping toxins that, as individuals, we can actually do very little to avoid. And I read that those fertility-zapping toxins weren't just in processed food and in its packaging materials. I read that they were in sanitary protection and in deodorants, in household cleaning products and in flame retardant sofa fillings, in the fumes from traffic and from industry and from pollution that we are constantly breathing in and that we are constantly – and frequently, inadvertently – ingesting in our food and in our drinking water.

I did know that it was unrealistic to aim to be living a 100 per cent toxin-free life in light of all of the environmental nasties that were floating about in our so-called developed world. So I decided to make a conscious effort not to worry about the myriad of fertility-impacting elements of modern life that I couldn't personally avoid, that I couldn't personally change. I had always had my doubts about the health-giving properties of caffeine, though, and of coffee in particular.

I had heard about a report that suggested there was a link between even the most moderate of intakes of caffeine and a greater risk of miscarriage. And so I decided to put two and two together. Okay, maybe I had put two and two together and come up with five. Maybe caffeine didn't have a negative impact on fertility. But I decided to make the change anyway, pre-emptively, before I managed to get pregnant. I switched to herbal teas, cutting right back on my tea and coffee consumption, thinking that if in some small way I could improve my general health by doing that then maybe, by association, I just might be able to improve my fertility too.

And I had heard that the consumption of alcohol wasn't particularly great news for fertility, either. For men – the small problem of brewers' droop put firmly to one side – I had heard that even the smallest amounts of alcohol could reduce sperm quantity and quality. And, for women, I had heard that alcohol could disrupt hormone levels, making it more difficult to get pregnant in the first place but then increasing the likelihood of miscarriages and of birth defects if a pregnancy *did* occur. I had heard that alcohol consumption could have a detrimental effect on the body's absorption of nutrients from food, too. And, now that I had started to hand over a small fortune for organic groceries every week, that was absolutely the last thing that I wanted.

So I all but eliminated alcohol from my own diet and, somehow, I managed to persuade Paul to reduce his alcohol consumption too, to restrict his drinking to weekends.

I must admit that it was easier for me. Since we had started trying for our baby, I had spent close to two weeks out of every month praying and hoping and, to be honest, semi-convinced that I was pregnant. And so consequently, for half of almost every month, for well over two years, I hadn't drunk anything alcoholic at all. The imagined and projected guilt of being responsible for foetal alcohol syndrome in my unborn (and, as it turned out month after month after month, un-conceived) child was more than I could have coped with. I even felt guilty if I ate blue cheese in the second half of my cycle – just on the off chance that I was carrying a tiny dot of a human being, the beginning of a baby in my womb who might have had an adverse reaction to the unpasteurized dairy product. And that's not to mention the jitteriness that came over me when I was exposed to the dangers of dippy eggs and other people's cigarettes, peanuts and pâté. And so cutting out even the occasional glass of white wine really did seem like a piece of cake.

What about Adoption?

'What *about* adoption?' After a couple of beers with our Friday night curry, Paul was expansive and open to the world of possibility.

'I don't know, I really don't.' My rogan josh washed down with nothing more potent than organic lemonade, I was feeling more practical. 'I worry about bonding. With your own – *natural* – child, I suppose you have had nine months' of practice at bonding before it's even born. What happens if it's more difficult to bond with an adopted child? What happens if it takes you longer to *love* them? Wouldn't they have had enough to deal with already? Wouldn't they have had enough trauma in their short lives – without finding themselves lumbered with an adoptive parent who was struggling to bond with them?'

'I suppose so,' Paul paused. 'But then you loved the *cat* instantly; you bonded with her as soon as we got her. And she's not even the same *species*.'

Paul did have a point but I still couldn't help having mixed feelings about adoption. I did remember a conversation that I'd had with a colleague. I remembered her telling me about her husband's very *positive* experience of being adopted.

'He found out when he was about five. His mum, the woman who'd adopted him, didn't want to leave it *too* long.

She didn't want him to find out about it from someone else.'

'God, he must have been devastated. When he did find out.'

'He wasn't, not really. His adoptive parents are just so lovely. And he remembers them handling it all really well. They told him that they hadn't been able to have children of their own and that they thought of him as a very special gift. They told him that he was an incredibly precious little boy and that they both loved him very much.'

'Amazing.'

'I suppose it was. I remember him telling me that he couldn't wait to get in to school the next day, the day after he'd found out. He couldn't wait to tell all of his friends about it.'

'Wow. Did he find out why had she given him up, his birth mother?'

'He did. It was the usual kind of thing, I suppose. His birth mother was just a kid herself. A very young, single girl who really didn't think that she could cope with raising a small child on her own.'

'Did he ever get in touch with her?'

'He did. But it wasn't until years later, not until he was well into his thirties. In fact it wasn't until we'd started thinking about having kids of our own. I think he'd wanted her to tie up a few loose ends for him. I think he'd wanted her to answer a few of the questions that his adoptive mother couldn't. They have met a couple of times since; she's got three other kids now. She'll never be able to take the place of his adoptive mother, though. His adoptive mother will always be 'mum' as far as he's concerned. And she'll always be grandma, too, as far as our kids are concerned.'

But then I had seen an item on the news about a couple who were attempting to sue their local council for not telling them that the child that they had adopted was seriously mentally disturbed, for not preparing them for the devastating consequences of having that particular child in their life. And I remembered reading somewhere that the development of children is in two key stages – between the ages of when they are born and three, and between the ages of three and six – and that if children are emotionally damaged during those formative years then they are basically screwed up for life. And, anyway, I had been told that you weren't allowed to apply to adopt a child until you could prove that you were no longer trying for your own.

Parsley, Sage, Rosemary and ... Agnus Castus?

The month after we had decided to put our fertility treatment on hold for the foreseeable future – and my first drug-free, first Clomid-free cycle for seven months – I was absolutely delighted when I spotted all of my usual ovulation indicators on exactly the day that I was expecting them. At the back of my mind I had had this annoyingly persistent worry that maybe it would take months for my hormone levels to get back to normal. I had read that for some women who had stopped taking the contraceptive pill in order to get pregnant, it had taken years. At least, I wanted to get back to what was normal for me. Happily, I quickly felt as though my body was my own again. And, with my new and improved diet – alcohol free and caffeine reduced – it was starting to feel like a far healthier and far more vibrant body than it had done for a very long time.

I was still aware, though, that even with the best and the freshest and the most balanced diet in the world, it could be difficult to get all of the nutrients and vitamins and minerals that the body needs for absolutely *optimum* health from food alone. And so my Internet browser took yet another battering as I began my on-line search for food supplements that would not only help me to improve my general health but would help me to boost my fertility, too.

I had never quite appreciated before the completely bewildering variety of vitamins and minerals that one was able to buy on the Internet. Many of them and particularly the ones that were reputed to have fertility-boosting properties I had never even *heard* of before. Some of the supplements were exclusively for men; still others were exclusively for women. Some of the supplements were exclusively for breast-feeding women, still others for menopausal women and for premenstrual women. It seemed that there was a food supplement to cover every possible demographic. Luckily, one of the on-line health food shops that my search engine had helped me to track down stocked a fairly comprehensive multivitamin that seemed to cover pretty much all of the bases for general and for reproductive health. There was one daily tablet for Paul and a different one for me. And so I added a couple of months' supply of each to my shopping basket.

The name of an herbal remedy kept cropping up in my on-line searches, too. An herbal remedy called Agnus Castus. Also known as Vitex. Also known as Chaste Tree Berry. And whatever its name, the more I read about it, the more the herbal remedy began to seem like something close to a wonder herb for women; to seem like something close to a cure-all. I read that Agnus Castus was reputed to be able to stimulate the function of the pituitary gland that could then, in turn, restore feminine hormonal balance to its optimum and natural state. Balancing out any excesses or deficiencies of oestrogen or progesterone. Helping to make periods more regular and less painful and less heavy. And – this was the part where my interest had really become piqued – helping infertile women to become pregnant. I guess it pretty much goes without saying that, before I had left that particular on-line health food shop, I had added a year's supply of Agnus Castus to my virtual shopping basket, too.

You're Back in the Room Now ...'

One morning, a close friend of mine who was, by that time, a mother of three had somehow managed to snatch five minutes for herself with some daytime television and a coffee. And, as luck would have it, she had caught the last few minutes of a feature about alternative therapies, a feature about a celebrity hypnotherapist who claimed to be able to help women who had been struggling to get pregnant, to help couples who had been diagnosed with unexplained infertility. And, immediately, my friend had thought about Paul and me and about what we were going through.

I was at work that day and by the time my thoughts had started turning toward lunch, my friend had called the TV show's health hotline, managed to get hold of the name and contact details of a hypnotherapist who practised in our local area and specialized in the treatment of infertility, and emailed the whole lot across to me. And so all that remained for me to do was to pick up the telephone. Lunchtime was the one and only time that our marketing office was pretty much guaranteed to be deserted. So that day, instead of joining my colleagues in the canteen for our usual office politics round up, I decided to give my local hypnotherapist a call.

I made the call and ended up chatting to the hypnotherapist for close to an hour. It really did feel as though a whole new world was being opened up to me. And one that seemed to make so much sense, one that seemed so kind of *obvious*. The hypnotherapist explained to me about the incredible power that the mind can have over the body. She explained to me that our minds on both a conscious and an unconscious level can have a strong influence on the physical symptoms that we experience in our bodies. She explained that everything we see and everything we hear and everything we experience is stored away somewhere within our bodies. She told me that these things could be stored away as memories or as beliefs, as emotions or as feelings, as dreams or as thoughts. And she told me that sometimes we are not even consciously aware of them. That sometimes they are locked away deep within us, in our unconscious mind, to protect us. But she explained to me that no matter how deeply buried those things were, they were still there, they were still powerful and they were still influential.

The hypnotherapist told me that it wasn't beyond the realms of possibility that my ability to conceive had been negatively affected by what other people had told me. What my friends had told me about the pain that they had experienced during the birth of their own children, for example, or what they had told me about the sheer physical exhaustion that they had experienced when caring for their newborn babies. And the hypnotherapist told me that my ability to conceive could have been negatively affected by my own thoughts, too, and by my own beliefs. She explained to me that many women have been telling themselves for years that the time – for a baby – is not quite right. And she told me that the same thing might well have been the case for me. She told me that that message might have still been getting through, even though on a conscious level I had made the decision that the time *was* right for Paul and me to have a baby.

And the hypnotherapist talked about how stress could have a negative impact on fertility, too. She told me that she understood just how very stressful the whole experience of trying for a baby can turn out to be; especially when it has been a long time, especially when medical assistance has had to be sought, especially when hopes are beginning to be dashed. And she told me that hypnotherapy could help to reduce that stress; that hypnotherapy could offer a particularly deep form of relaxation, helping to remove old emotional blocks, to improve mental and physical and spiritual well-being. And she told me that she had produced a CD, to help women like me, to help couples like us.

Opening Pandora's Box

I ordered the *Hypnotherapy for Fertility* CD immediately. Trying to persuade Paul to listen to the CD with me took a little longer. He was certainly sceptical, and I think he may even have been a little bit scared. A little bit scared that hypnotherapy was yet another one of the supposedly sure-fire solutions that I seemed to want to cling on to, that I seemed to *need* to cling on to, like a life raft in our sea of involuntary childlessness.

'Are you sure that this isn't just another one of your trying-for-a-baby bandwagons? We've tried fertility drugs and IUI. We've cut back on alcohol and caffeine and processed food. You're still seeing your homeopath and taking that multivitamin and that herbal remedy …' Paul softened, 'Look, I'm just worried that if you don't get the outcome that you want …'

'The outcome that *both* of us want!'

'OK, OK. I'm just worried that you're going to end up disappointed, that we're *both* going to end up disappointed. When we made the decision to stop fertility treatment for a bit, it felt as though we had got our life back again. It felt as though we had put the baby thing into perspective. But now it seems as though it's all that we ever talk about. Again. And I'm really worried that it's all that you ever *think* about.'

The concept of separate realities is certainly a strange one. Paul's reality seemed to be that we never stopped talking about trying for a baby; my reality was that we hardly *ever* talked about it and that we certainly didn't talk about it enough. But I knew that, in one way, he was right. I *was* always thinking about babies. I was prepared to try absolutely anything that I thought might help us to have one. And anything that didn't involve fertility drugs and hormonal disruption, invasive medical procedures and appointments with fertility specialists seemed to me to be well worth a go.

The first time that I listened to the CD, I was astounded. Long-since-forgotten comments from my friends and my family just seemed to pop into my mind, as fresh and as clear as if I had heard them yesterday. I couldn't believe just how many negative messages I had absorbed and internalized over the years. So many negative messages concerning getting pregnant, about giving birth, about raising children, about becoming a mother. And the negative messages were not just confined to real life memories. I recalled things that I had read in books and in magazines, things that I had seen on TV and in films. Years before. Long since forgotten. It seemed as though every single negative comment that I had ever heard about having babies came flooding right back into my conscious mind.

Messages such as, 'Once you have been pregnant, once you have had a child, you can kiss goodbye to ever feeling sexy or ever feeling desirable again'. Messages like, 'Once you have had children, you *will* get fat, without a shadow of a doubt. Your figure will never be the same again. There will be cellulite and stretch marks, not to mention the jangled nerves and the bags under your eyes'. Messages like, 'In the extremely unlikely event that your partner still finds you attractive – and hasn't run off with his sexy and young and *child-free* business associate, he will eventually get frustrated by your constant exhaustion, by your lack of interest in him. He will become increasingly jealous and resentful of the child that has become the centre of your universe'.

And – in return for the sacrifices of your looks and your relationship, in return for your round-the-clock devotion – your child will do nothing but scream through the night. It will scream through most of the day, too. It will drain you of your energy. It will drain you of your youth. It will drain you of your money. You could buy yourself a Porsche, apparently, if you didn't have to stump up for disposable nappies and for school shoes and the very latest in Japanese pre-school toy trends. And one message was loud and clear – you might as well forget about your career. That was unless you particularly wanted your children to resent you for the rest of your life and theirs – because you were so incredibly selfish as to choose to work rather than be with them. And, anyway, working mothers were evil. Everyone knew that. It didn't matter what you did though, at the end of the day, it didn't matter how many sacrifices you made. Your kids would resent you anyway and blame you and sneer at you and maybe even despise you. They would resent you for not being rich enough or cool enough. They would resent you for being too rich or for being too cool.

And, fairly unsurprisingly, none of those messages was doing a particularly good job of selling motherhood to me. And those messages were just the very tip of a whole iceberg of negativity that I uncovered using my *Hypnotherapy for Fertility* CD.

Digging a Little Deeper

I started to remember specific incidents, too, and with an incredible and almost startling clarity. I remembered how we had rushed along to the maternity ward of our local hospital to welcome a friend's newborn daughter into the world. And how, when I had held her, the baby had cried. I remembered my friend saying, 'That's the first time she's ever cried.' And although I knew that my initial, almost instinctive reply of, 'Oh well, I'm pretty sure that it won't be the last time!' was a logical one and a sensible one, somehow I had managed to internalize a very different message – an unbelievably negative one. That message was, 'See, you can't even hold a baby for five minutes without making her cry. It's probably just as well that you can't have kids of your own. You don't have a maternal bone in your body. You would be a terrible mother. You would be a dreadful mother.'

And I remembered that the guys where I used to work had had a '*Top Totty?*' list. Rumour had it that there was even a spreadsheet somewhere – on some enlightened soul's PC – so that the movers and the shakers, the winners and the losers in the office beauty queen stakes could be quickly and easily added to the list. Or just as quickly and easily deleted from it. I remember hearing how the 'Toppest of Totties' had been removed from the list altogether when she was 'unlucky' enough to get herself pregnant. And I remember feeling unsure about whether to be heartened by her removal from the list – by the almost chivalrous nature of my male colleagues that had seemed to say, 'Well, she's going to be a mum. She's definitely out of our league now' – or disheartened. Disheartened because as soon as that particular woman had conceived her first child, it seemed that she had automatically rendered herself absolutely unattractive to the opposite sex too.

And I remembered how I felt physically, when I let my own thinking become negative, when I let my own thinking become pessimistic. How as soon as I allowed myself to voice the words, even to myself, 'I am infertile, I will never have a baby', my entire body had seemed to become leaden and heavy, my entire body had seemed to sigh with defeat. I thought about the label that had been applied to Paul and me, too. About our diagnosis of infertility – unexplained infertility, but infertility nonetheless. And I thought about just how desperate and sad, how pointless and pitiful that had made me feel. I thought about all of the negative and almost doom-laden messages that I had taken on board about fertility over the years, too. About time running out, for women, once they had hit their thirties. About conception opportunities dwindling rapidly and about the likelihood for miscarriage and for birth defects increasing dramatically.

And, for the first time, I began to appreciate the incredible power that the mind can have over the healthy functioning, or otherwise, of the body. And, somehow, it didn't seem quite so surprising any more that my mind hadn't been giving my body the right messages in order for me to become pregnant. And incredibly, and despite all of the negative thoughts and feelings that had risen up to the surface, after listening to the *Hypnotherapy for Fertility* CD I felt amazing. Really positive and light and totally convinced that my body *did* know how to get pregnant – deep down – and that, eventually, I *would* get pregnant, in my own good time.

Racing through the Best Days

It's strange, really, how it's often the most seemingly inconsequential events that become the catalysts for the major decisions in our lives, for the really life-changing ones. I remember an old work colleague – and someone who I actually respected and valued as a person and as a friend – returning to the office after a day away at one of those empowering, feel-good, executive-type conferences. The kind of thing that savvy companies send their employees to, intermittently, to make them think, 'This company isn't such a bad place to work after all. We get to have whole days away from the office. We get to go on inspirational courses'. (And then those savvy companies can get away without giving pay rises to their staff for yet another year. But that's another long and boring story.)

Bubbling over with optimism after her day out of the office – perhaps unsurprising since the two were, often, not unrelated factors – initially, my colleague's enthusiasm had been contagious, as she had relayed golden nuggets of wisdom from the plethora of engaging and motivational speakers that she had seen the day before. And then she started telling me about an incredible development in time management that she had heard about. She started telling me about Quantum Reading.

About how you could absorb the contents of an entire book simply by holding the book's spine, flicking through the pages and letting your eyes just drift over the words. And that all you had to do was make an affirmation at the start, along the lines of: 'OK. I'm going to learn all that there is to know about international branding strategy or brain surgery or what happens in the latest Harry Potter' – or whatever the book happened to be about. The fact of the matter was that you could absorb the contents of a *whole book* in a matter of minutes. It seemed that all the high achievers were using the technique, all the corporate big hitters.

At first I thought that the technique sounded incredible, that Quantum Reading sounded amazing. And I must admit that my mind went into overdrive, mentally listing all of the books that I would dearly love to read but had, somehow, never quite found the time. All of those newly released contemporary novels; and all of the classics, too. All of those life improving self-help books. Never mind all of the tedious work-related publications that I never seemed to be able to muster the energy or the inclination to plough through. But then I started to think, *hang on a minute, this is a world gone mad.* Why can't we just set aside an hour or so to enjoy the experience of reading? Why does life have to be raced through quantumly or otherwise? A small, somewhat inconvenient, hurdle like reading easily overcome ... And, when I thought a little bit harder, I started to realize that I was already applying this quantum approach to almost every aspect of my life.

I would eat out or buy takeaways or use pre-prepared M&S ingredients – organic mind you – because there never seemed to be enough time to shop, let alone to cook. And I had always loved poring over recipe books and planning menus. I had always loved cooking.

I would let expensive tour operators worry about my holiday destinations and organize my travel itineraries because I never seemed to be able to find the time to just open an atlas, to just spin a globe and see what far-flung place took my fancy. And my time away from work was so very precious to me.

I was prepared to hand over my hard earned cash to pay for a cleaner, to pay for a gardener. Because the more money I earned, the less time I seemed to have to do my own cleaning, to do my own gardening. And I found both activities calming; I found both therapeutic.

And when I took an even longer, even harder look at my life I had just one thought. *That it had become like madness.* That it had become like absolute madness.

Golden Handcuffs

I suppose that we had been lucky Paul and me – in so many different ways. We felt blessed that we had found each other, that we had got together – soul mates, two sides of the same coin – while we were still in our early twenties; years before we saw friends of ours, pushing thirty and frantic because they *still* hadn't tracked down Mr or Ms Right.

And good fortune had seemed to smile on us at work, too. Paul and I had both always seemed to be in the right place at the right time when promotions and pay rises were being handed out. And we had both switched companies a few times, taking advantage of the fact that the new company will rarely pay you less than the old one. We had also struck it lucky with property, managing to sell the first house that we had bought together, in a suddenly sought-after part of town, for a fairly substantial profit. And I suppose that that should have been a warning bell for us, really. It should have been a wake-up call.

We had both always said that as soon as we had got a decent amount of money together, we would pack in our jobs and do something different – we would really 'live' our life. I had always wanted to write, to try my hand at becoming a novelist. Paul had often talked about us buying a tumbling-down wreck, somewhere romantically remote, and about us getting freelance work or even bar jobs to fund the bits of the renovation that we couldn't do ourselves. Most importantly, though, we had planned to spend lots of time together – huge chunks of quality time. But somewhere along the line we had both seemed to forget about really living our life.

Maybe my career had been at some excitingly crucial point. Or maybe it was Paul's. Maybe we had been at a stage where the trappings of our increasingly work-oriented lives – two respectable incomes, two company cars and plenty of spare cash – had just seemed to be too difficult to walk away from. Whatever. The 'really living our life' thing just didn't happen. We ended up using the profit from the sale of our first house as down payment on another one. On a house that was bigger and better and more expensive. And, in the blink of an eye, it seemed as though we had committed ourselves to living exactly the kind of lives that when we had first got together, we had sworn that we never would. We were living to work instead of working to live. We were stressing over the minutiae, like work deadlines and office politics, mortgage repayments and pension schemes. We forgot to clock off. We started bringing our work home. And over the years – with the new jobs and the pay rises and the promotions – it gradually felt as though we had lost sight of our dreams.

I used to try to tell myself that things would change when I got pregnant, when Paul and I had had our first baby. I would work part-time, then. Maybe I would give up work altogether. And then our life could start to revolve around our home instead of our offices. Our life could revolve around our family. It could revolve around us. And I remember having this expectation that, when Paul and I had had a baby, everything about our life would be different. Everything about our life would be better. Everything would be more real. And maybe that was part of the problem. Maybe my expectations were too high, for our unborn child. Maybe my expectations were too high for a child that seemed incredibly reluctant to be conceived.

Sticking a Pin in a Map of the World

There is a certain sense of irony, I suppose, that because of the way our life had unfolded, in the end it was our *not* having a baby that changed everything for us. Because achieving a pregnancy had continued to elude us – and because Paul and Isla still only had Paul and Isla to worry about – we both realized that we had some breathing space for ourselves. We realized that we had a golden opportunity. An opportunity to actually *listen* to some of those wake-up calls that had seemed to keep telling us – quietly but insistently – that our life wasn't all it could be, our life wasn't all it *should* be. And we realized that not only could we listen to those wake-up calls but that we could act on them too. We realized that we had the freedom to change our life, together, into whatever we wanted it to be.

And so we talked about all of the life changes we *could* make. About all of the little things we could do to make our life better. I said that I would like to reduce the number of hours that I spent at work, that I would like to spend more time working at home, maybe, that I would like to consider working part-time. I even talked about the possibility of working in a completely different industry. I talked about the possibility of retraining – training to become a counsellor, maybe, or a psychotherapist. Something that felt more worthwhile, more rewarding than my job in marketing. And Paul talked about some ideas that he had had for a business of his own and he started to sound more excited about the prospect of work than he had done in years.

And then we talked about the possibility of selling our house. House prices in our area had rocketed and so we had the option of selling our house and cashing in on its equity, we had the option of trading in the old place for something smaller and something cheaper.

And then the realization slowly dawned on both of us that the life changes that we made didn't have to be small. The life changes that we made could be massive. They could be as monumental as we wanted them to be. We could sell our house. We could leave our jobs, too. We could have a completely fresh start. We could live a totally different life. And we could do all of it somewhere new. And, after the emotional turmoil of everything that we had been through, the idea of a fresh start appealed to both of us. So selling our house and leaving our jobs and starting afresh was exactly what we decided to do.

I suppose that, like many people, Paul and I had had the occasional eliminatory discussions about where, in an ideal world, we would like to live. The discussions were usually fuelled by a couple of glasses of wine and the prospect of having to get up for work the next morning and so, up until that point, our discussions had been based on pipe dreams. When we could fondly imagine that money was not and never would be an object. When we could dream about spending our days strolling idly along endless sun-drenched and palm-fringed tropical beaches. But Paul and I had moved on from pipe dreams. And now we needed to try and narrow down the whole wide world into the perfect relocation location. We needed to find somewhere we could both realistically and happily live and, ultimately, work. And the world had, all of a sudden, started to seem as though it was a very big place.

We both loved Australia. Paul had always said that he would move there in a flash. But for me, a girl who had never even moved out of Yorkshire, Australia seemed as though it was just one step too far. Australia seemed too final, somehow. And, if I am being honest, I think that I was scared of kissing such a significant goodbye to my relationships with my family and my friends. Scared of finding out just how many of those relationships would fall by the wayside if I relocated to the other side of the world. And so we turned our attention to places that were a little bit closer to home. We turned our attention to the European stars of the countless relocation TV shows – to Spain and to France and to Italy. And, at first, both of us were incredibly tempted.

'Any of those places would be gorgeous. Just think about all of that fresh, locally produced food. Think about the wine …'

'Think about the weather; long, hot summers, swimming in the sea, barbecues in the back garden …'

'And barbecues in the back garden of a house that had cost us practically *nothing.*'

It was me who had chosen to burst our Mediterranean bubble:

'I suppose that it might be a bit hard to get settled in, though. Not speaking the language. My French is as rusty as anything. And if we *do* struggle with the language, it might make it difficult for us to get work, when the house funds run out …'

And so we had turned our thoughts even *closer* to home. We had started to think about Ireland and – for both of us – Ireland just seemed so obvious. My grandfather had been born in a village just outside Dublin. Most of Paul's family was still living in Northern Ireland. And so the whole *concept* of moving to the Republic of Ireland, to the Emerald Isle, just felt like moving home. We were seduced by the thought of Ireland's legendary hospitality, by the thought of the chilled-out people who enjoyed a slower pace of life and who still had time for each other. We were attracted to Ireland's sense of history and of culture and of the arts. We felt drawn to Ireland's scenery, from its rugged and breathtakingly beautiful coastlines to its bustling little market towns. And the more we talked about Ireland, the closer our minds were to being made up.

'Much Sought after'?

We thought that it would probably be a good idea to *visit* Ireland to make absolutely sure that the reality of the place lived up to our fond imaginings. So we decided to book ourselves an exploratory week's holiday. We thought that a week would give us just enough time to get a feel for the place, just enough time to check out the local property market.

And, since we knew that, that week was really going to fly past, we thought that it would be a good idea to try and pull some sort of plan together, so that we could really make the most of our trip. So, before we left, we pored over a growing pile of guidebooks in an attempt to compile a short-list of some description, an attempt to pull together a list of counties to investigate properly while we were in Ireland. This, in itself, turned out to be no mean feat. We didn't have much to go on, to be honest – just a combination of the vague, tourist-centric and rather brief descriptions from our guidebooks and Paul's somewhat rudimentary knowledge of the Republic of Ireland's geography.

Helpfully, one particular county discounted itself almost automatically after we had read, in our trusty guidebooks, about its occupants having a higher than usual propensity for getting themselves shot or stabbed – a violent prospect that wasn't entirely in keeping with our rose-tinted preconception of life in a rural idyll. And we knew that we wanted to live near the sea, and so that helped us to narrow down our list of potential counties a little bit further. And then, after somewhat arbitrarily discounting all of the other counties – as too expensive or too flat, as too industrial or too land bound, as too *something* that wasn't quite right – we eventually came up with our hot list of counties. We decided to focus our attention on counties Cork, Kerry, Galway and Clare. And we decided to have a quick look on the Internet to see what house prices were like in those counties, to see what kind of places were for sale.

The downright honesty of the Irish property particulars, especially when compared to the flowery descriptions that I had got used to hearing from English estate agents amazed me. When we had bought one of our houses in England, I remember the lounge being described as 'benefiting from an understairs study area'. That 'understairs study area' had later become a shoe cupboard and that gives some indication of the size of the space that we are talking about. And as fond as I am of shoes, I am certainly no Imelda Marcos. On the Irish property websites, instead of the descriptions of 'charming country lanes' that we had come to expect from English estate agents, we read about 'ruinous cottages situated miles along dirt tracks'. And instead of 'delightful properties that were in need of some modernization', we read about 'buildings that were in a very poor state of repair and that would, ideally, need to be knocked down in order to build a new dwelling'.

The Irish estate agents certainly didn't mince their words. And it was incredibly refreshing and, frequently, entertaining to read about houses 'that were basically a collection of stone ruins which dated back to the famine period' and 'that were last used as a home for cattle so absolutely everything needed to be done in order to make them habitable'.

Paul and I giggled together about the typos, about the spelling mistakes and about the general inconsistencies in the Irish property descriptions. Some properties would have their selling prices quoted in euros. Some in pounds; some would have their selling prices quoted in dollars; some even in the long defunct punts. And, rather confusingly, some properties on the same estate agent's books would have their selling prices quoted in a combination of all four of the currencies but – to add to the general sense of confusion – never in quite the same order. I could vividly imagine the pedant in some middle England estate agent's office, presiding with anal retention over brochure production. 'No, no, no Miss Smith – pounds sterling and *then* euros, with three spaces separating the two and the euros value always bracketed.'

I positively drooled over charming little hand-drawn maps. The key landmarks seemed to be more about quaintly named pubs and local stores, more about village post offices and riding stables than about motorway junctions and A-roads, or house numbers and twenty-four hour petrol stations. And I let my imagination run wild over evocative directions that seemed to be all about windy roads and grottoes and white and cream farm houses with fuchsia hedges outside. Even phrases like, 'a well would need to be bored for water' and, 'a septic tank would have to be installed' couldn't put me off. And this was me who, just a year or two earlier, would have rejected a potential new house after one viewing on the basis that I didn't like the pattern on the tiles in the downstairs toilet.

I remember phoning an estate agent just before we arrived in County Kerry. I wanted to see how up to date their website was. I wanted to find out if a particularly gorgeous property – all tumbling down charm and stone outbuildings and acres and acres of land – that we had spotted on their website was still for sale. In England, we had had to get used to places being sold before their 'For Sale' was even stuck in the ground and neither of us wanted to fall in love with a photograph of a cottage only to find out that it had been sold months previously. When the phone was eventually answered – no procedure for answering within three rings – I described the property in question to the estate agent.

'Oh, it's still available,' I was told.

And I asked how long the cottage had been on the market for.

'Oh, years,' came the reply, giving me the distinct impression that it wasn't likely to be sold for years either, that I had all the time in the world. And I remember asking the guy in the estate agent's office if they opened seven days a week. I was trying to get some kind of plan in place, after all. I was trying to make sure that we made the most of our weeklong trip.

'God, no. Sure, aren't you long enough dead?'

And that was that. I, for one, had fallen for Ireland – hook, line and sinker.

Playing a Numbers Game

By the time that we had made up our minds to radically change our life – to leave our jobs and to sell our house and to relocate to the south of Ireland – Paul and I had been trying to have a baby together for just over three years. And, although maths had never been a particularly strong point of mine, my thoughts had turned to the numbers game that getting pregnant appeared to be. My thoughts had started to turn to luck and to probability and to chance. I do remember hearing somewhere that human beings, as a species, are just about the least fertile of mammals. And I remember hearing that, for us sub-fertile human beings, even if our reproductive equipment is in perfect working order and even if we manage to get the timing of our 'hoping-for-a-baby sex' absolutely right, there is still only a 20 per cent chance of us getting pregnant every month.

And my friend had told me that the window of opportunity for conception was, on average, a pretty measly two days each month. And even I could work out that that was just twenty-four days' worth of opportunities in an entire year.

Three years of trying for a baby had felt like a very long time. If I am being honest, three years of trying for a baby had felt like an absolute *lifetime*. But it didn't take a mathematical genius to calculate that – even over the three-year period that

Paul and I had been trying and hoping and praying to conceive – there had still been just a fairly paltry seventy-two days' worth of opportunities. And when I thought about it like that – when I looked at it logically, when I looked at it *statistically* – somehow it didn't seem quite so strange that I hadn't managed to get pregnant. I started to think that maybe Paul and I had just been unlucky. I was pretty sure that, on a good proportion of those seventy-two days, Paul and I hadn't been in the same place; that we hadn't even been in the same country. I was also sure that, on another good proportion of those seventy-two days, one or the other of us had been a bit tipsy or a bit run down or a bit stressed out – or maybe even a combination of all three – making our baby making bits function less than optimally. And maybe, on more occasions than we had realized, we just hadn't been in the mood.

And so, without becoming obsessive, Paul and I had refocused our efforts on doing whatever we could to improve our chances of having a baby, naturally. Our diet – fresh and unprocessed and organic – was already just about as healthy as it could be. I had been caffeine reduced and alcohol free for months. The prospect of leaving our jobs had made the stress of them disappear almost overnight. And taking Agnus Castus, the wonder herb for women, had become as natural a part of my morning routine as brushing my teeth. And so – to improve our odds still further in the numbers game that making a baby appeared to be – we decided to use a combination of what I had learned about the physical indications of ovulation and the good old-fashioned calendar method. We pinpointed my most fertile days and we made damn sure that we had sex on each and every one of them.

Waiting

As had so often seemed to be the case whenever we booked a holiday – whether it was for a fortnight, for a long weekend or even for just an overnight trip – I was expecting my period on the first day of our week in Ireland. On the very first day, the Monday, the day that we had planned to drive down to Wales, to hop on a ferry and then to drive the six or so hours across Ireland from Dublin's ferry port to County Kerry. And, quite naturally, I hadn't been entirely happy about the prospect of being cooped up in our car for hours on end with the type of painful stomach cramps that always accompanied the first day of my period, the type of painful stomach cramps that only ever seemed to be alleviated by physical activity, by moving around. And I wasn't exactly overjoyed about the prospect of having only intermittent access to toilet facilities either. But still, we carried on with our Irish fact-finding mission as planned.

Tuesday morning had found us installed in the centrally located, family run B&B and pub combo that we had chosen as our base for the week; refreshed after more than twelve hours of much needed sleep. And as yet there was no sign of anything, period-wise. At first, I tried to explain it away. I put it down to excitement about our Ireland trip. I dismissed it as a side effect of the Agnus Castus that I had been taking for the previous few months. I even thought that maybe it was just me, getting my dates muddled – uncharacteristically, admittedly. In the years that Paul and I had been trying for our baby I had learnt how to calculate my period due dates with an almost uncanny accuracy. And so we continued with our tour of as much of the South West of Ireland as it was humanly possible to cover. We took in quaint little market towns and dramatically windswept and deserted beaches; we took in picturesque streets lined with pastel-painted cottages. And we fell in love with Ireland.

By Wednesday night, my period still hadn't started and the suspense was close to killing me, the suspense was close to killing *both* of us. And I, for one, was finding it increasingly difficult to stop the tiniest little bit of excitement from creeping in.

'No PMT this month,' I ventured.

I could see Paul racking his brain, searching for examples of any typically period-onset behaviour that he could cite and, clearly, he was struggling to come up with any.

'Couldn't that be the Agnus Castus, though? Isn't that supposed to get rid of the symptoms of PMT? Isn't that supposed to make the second half of your cycle longer, too?'

I let this information sink in for a moment or two.

'You're right, it is. But I've been taking Agnus Castus for months. You would have thought that any changes that it was going to make would have settled down by now ... And, anyway, what about at my cousin's wedding? I couldn't face even a *sip* of champagne during the toasts ... And I left my after-dinner coffee.'

'Maybe you're just not used to the taste any more, of either of them. You haven't drunk any alcohol or any coffee for months.'

'Hmm, maybe ... I am really tired, though. Inexplicably so after the amount of sleep that we've both had over the last couple of days.' And I remember stretching and letting out a dramatically noisy yawn to illustrate my point.

I knew that it was time to put an end to the speculation and we both decided that, if nothing had happened overnight, we would buy a pregnancy test first thing next morning.

Little Blue Line

Thursday morning arrived as Thursday mornings do. And nothing *had* happened overnight. We wolfed down our breakfast and headed out to buy a pregnancy test from the local chemist. As we made our way back to our room in the B&B, I could feel my heart pounding. Almost sick with the sense of anticipation – not to mention the hastily eaten full Irish – I shut myself away in the en-suite. My heart plummeted from my mouth to my feet as a dark horizontal line instantly appeared in the test's result window. I had been there before; more times than I cared to remember during the three and a half years that Paul and I had been trying for our baby. We put the pregnancy test to one side, left it to develop for the required couple of minutes. And we waited. We shook our watches; we tapped their faces, thoroughly convinced that they must have both been running slow. And then the time was up.

I picked up the test and stared at it, probably open-mouthed. I couldn't believe my eyes. I shoved the test toward Paul. And I don't think that he could believe his eyes either. The test was positive. I was pregnant. We hugged and we kissed and we cried tears of absolute joy. I read and re-read the test's instruction leaflet, to make doubly sure, triply sure that there hadn't been some kind of mistake. Paul even took a photo of the pregnancy test's result window, with our digital camera. And, strangely, the image that I saw on the camera's tiny screen seemed much more real than what I could see in real life, right there in front of me. It is a truism, I suppose, that the camera never lies.

Paul and I were every single one and more of the happiness clichés – we were cock-a-hoop, we were over the moon, we were jumping for joy and we were, indeed, as happy as Larry. We were overjoyed that I was pregnant – just months after making the painful decision to leap off the fertility treatment conveyor belt. Just weeks after we had sold our house in England to carve out a new path for ourselves, in Ireland.

I don't think that I had ever before experienced such pure and intense and uncomplicated joy. I was going to have a baby with the man that I loved. I would be the mother of Paul's child. I would be someone's *mother*. We had created something beautiful together – Paul and me – something meaningful. We were going to be a family. That baby – our baby! – the first step toward the kind of noisy and boisterous and argumentative and *loving* family that I had always wanted for myself. And I was determined that I was going to be the best mum ever.

We thought that we would keep the news to ourselves, at first. That we would catch up with our family and with our close friends, in person, as soon as we got home. But both of us felt as though we were bursting with excitement and we decided that we would give our parents a quick call. And, OK then, our brothers. And then we decided to phone a few of our friends just the closest ones. And then that was it – the word was out.

The Best Laid Plans

We spent the rest of that week in Ireland floating around in our own blissful little bubble made for three. Everything we saw, every town and every street, every house and every person seemed absolutely delightful to me. And I knew, even then, that my observations were far from being objective but I was just too happy to care. How could I not fall head-over-heels in love with everything I saw and everything I experienced? Everything seemed to be bathed in such a positive light. Everything seemed to be almost inextricably linked to our own incredible news.

We had planned that when we got back from our Ireland trip, and the moment that the contracts on our house sale were finally and safely exchanged, I would resign. We had planned to put all of our belongings into storage and to stay in a spare room at my parents' house until my notice was served. I needed to give my company three months' notice. And three months had seemed as though it was a very long time when Paul and I had both been so impatient to be gone. When we had both been so impatient to be making a start on our new life.

But when we found out that I was pregnant, everything seemed to lose its sense of urgency. We even started to think about tweaking our plans a bit, in light of our newly changed circumstances. We thought that if I carried on working for just three months longer than we had originally planned – a period of time that, all of a sudden, seemed like a drop in the ocean over the course of a lifetime – I would be able to go on maternity leave. I would be able to take advantage of a full year off work – complete with benefits like pension payments, a fully financed company car and weeks and weeks of holidays in lieu. We could still stay at my mum and dad's house for a bit but just until we had found somewhere that we could rent in England for twelve months or so. And then, when my maternity leave was up, I could just change my mind about returning to work and we could pick up with our Ireland plans almost exactly where we had left off – just one year later and with our brand new baby on board.

And, anyway, we thought that we had plenty of time in which to make up our minds.

One of Life's Most Stressful Experiences?

I certainly wasn't unhappy to be leaving our house in England, to be selling up – quite the opposite, in a lot of ways. In fact I can remember feeling a quite distinct sense of relief. I think I had started to associate the house itself, perhaps somewhat unfairly, with a certain amount of unhappiness.

We had lived in that house for a couple of years. And, during the time that we had been there, Paul had gradually become more and more disillusioned with his job and with his career. Both of us had faced a couple of years of insecurity, a couple of years of uncertainty, as Paul had jumped from role to role, from company to company, from industry to industry – in search of a sense of happiness, a sense of fulfilment that was to remain elusive for him. In the year or so before we had made the decision to move to Ireland, each of Paul's roles at work had turned out to be just as unfulfilling for him as the one that had gone before.

'I think I would feel differently if we had kids,' Paul had once told me, 'If we had kids, I would feel as though I had something to work *for*.' And I knew how he felt.

Because, of course, we had had the sadness of our involuntary childlessness to deal with. Our friends had conceived and given birth to first and second and third babies while Paul and I had lived in that house. And we had both experienced a very real sense of loneliness as our friends' lives had necessarily become more inward facing and more family focused, just when our lives – for the sake of our own sanity – had been crying out for help and for reassurance and for, well, friendship.

It had seemed like a long time since I had thought of that house of ours as a home. I think as soon as we had made the decision to sell the place, to move to Ireland, all those weeks before, the house had become nothing more than a roof over our heads. And the house was starting to display signs of that emotional abandonment; it was starting to display signs of neglect. Almost as soon as we had put our house on the market, any housework had been either a cursory nod toward a basic level of hygiene or carried out in a mad flurry of air freshener and furniture polish just moments before a potential buyer was due to arrive. Not to mention the indefinite postponement of any non-essential DIY projects. Unless it was something that could actually deter a buyer, something that could affect the asking price, it just didn't get done.

When we had moved into that particular house, Paul and I had both thought that we would be there for a good few years. We had fully expected that that would be the house where we would have our children, that that would become our first family home. The house had an enormous loft, one of the things that had really sold the place to us – a loft that had been ripe for conversion into acres of play area for the houseful of kids that we had both dreamed about. A loft that could even have been turned into a chill-out area for the happily frazzled mum and dad of our imaginations.

On the day that we moved out, that loft was still just a rather cobwebby storage area. I think I would have found that more difficult to deal with if I hadn't been pregnant. I think I would have struggled to deal with the significance of what that vast, empty space represented. That despite all of our plans and our hopes and our dreams, that loft, our family space, was still untouched. But I *was* pregnant. And so I didn't think that I had to worry too much about metaphors.

The Beginning of ...

As much as I love my mum and dad, I had certainly never imagined that in my early thirties, I would be at home living with them. I never imagined that I would be living there, with a husband and a cat in tow, and with a baby on the way. I would have never imagined that the very few clothes that Paul and I had chosen not to sell at car boot sales would be hanging in the wardrobe in my parents' spare room. That the few belongings that we had thought that we really couldn't live without would be in cardboard boxes in my parents' garage. And for the first couple of weeks that we were living there, life couldn't have been better.

Our cat lost no time at all in making herself at home, taking every advantage of the novelty of fully stocked and regularly replenished food cupboards. And, to be honest, so did Paul and I. Filling our boots with three square meals and home grown vegetables and freshly baked bread and delicious cakes and general, well, scrumminess. Incredibly quickly, the pair of us adapted to our new life of absolutely no responsibility. Not having to check if the doors were locked or if the windows were shut or if the gas was off. Not having to worry about food shopping or mortgage repayments or overlooked bills. The first week that Paul and I spent at my mum and dad's house was one of total relaxation, one of absolute bliss. And that cocoon of comfort, that cocoon of homeliness went some way toward distracting me from what was going on at work.

Our department was going through a comprehensive restructuring programme that was, somewhat predictably, becoming rather painful. The wild speculation, the impromptu meetings to discuss the latest version of, 'You'll never guess what I saw on the photocopier …', the rapidly increasing certainty of a future – smaller – department full of hurt feelings and dented egos. Looking back, I don't really understand how I let myself become so emotionally involved, so tangled up in it all. It was a show of solidarity, I suppose, for my colleagues – for people with whom I spent most of my waking hours. I was railing against the unfairness of what seemed to be happening to them. Because unless I was made redundant – redundancy and pregnancy being two extremely highly charged words when it came to unfair dismissal tribunals – the restructure couldn't really affect me. Not personally. I planned to be out of the company within a year anyway, to be swapping a life of corporate manoeuvres and office politics for one of creativity and home making. And for becoming a mother ...

... The Middle of ...

I had never been quite so glad for a working week to be over as I was that particular week. It seemed as though every single person in the department was involved in the increasingly heated and fraught and feverish predictions over the outcome of the restructure. No one wanted to talk about anything else. It felt as though there was no respite. And on the journey home to my parents' house on that Friday night, I felt as though the vicarious emotional turmoil of the week was finally starting to catch up with me. I felt awful. And I put it down to the horrendous week that I had just endured; a couple of hours stuck on the motorway, in rush hour traffic, on what surely must have been the hottest and stickiest day of the summer being the cherry on the top of a particularly unpalatable cake.

When I arrived at my parents' house wrung out and absolutely exhausted, I found it impossible to concentrate hard enough or long enough to have anything more than a perfunctory conversation with my mum. I just about managed to convey my desire for a long soak in the bath before dragging myself off, up the stairs. I do remember seeing a small darkish patch, glistening damply, as I stepped out of my black underwear. It didn't look like blood, though. And the warm scented bubbles of my bath quickly and effectively washed away any sense of concern that I might otherwise have had. And then I had a ridiculously early night. Effortlessly drifting off to sleep to the uncomplicatedly happy sounds of the neighbour's young children, still playing together outside, taking full advantage of the warmth and light of the evening ...

'You know that dark stuff that I was telling you about? I'm still getting it. I think there's quite a bit more of it today, though.'

'Is it blood? Are you worried about it?'

'No and well ... No. Not really. But I think I just need some-body else to tell me that it's nothing to worry about.'

'Phone NHS Direct, then and see what they reckon.'

I did call NHS Direct. And they reckoned that there probably wasn't too much for me to worry about. *Blood* was what I did need to worry about – fresh, bright, red blood. And so I was OK then.

It was a much cooler day and so we decided to head out for a walk (Paul and me) in an attempt to blow away a few of the cobwebs after being cooped up in our respectively hot and sticky offices all week. When we got back to my mum and dad's house, I slept for a couple of hours, mindful of a night out that I had arranged with Paul and a couple of workmates. Mindful of a night out that I was still fully intending to enjoy.

The four of us headed out to a local gastro-pub. We bought a round of drinks – Paul exploiting the fact that, for the next seven months at least, I would definitely be driving – and, after some enjoyable deliberation about a comprehensively delicious menu, we put in our food orders. I headed off to find the toilet, then. I had felt a kind of sticky dampness and wanted to check that, whatever it was, it was still darkish and not the fresh, bright, red blood that the NHS Direct person had told me to watch out for. But there it was. Fresh. Bright. Red. Blood. Just a drop or two of it, but fresh, bright, red blood nonetheless. I didn't know what to do. I didn't want to be overly dramatic – cutting short the evening because of a drop of blood in my knickers. And so I opted, at first, for the burying-my-head-in-the-sand strategy.

I joined the others, attempting to shoehorn myself into their already lively conversation. But my heart just wasn't in it. My thoughts kept darting back to that fresh, bright, red blood – to the implications of it. At the time, I remember hoping – I remember praying – that I was just being paranoid. I remember bargaining with myself, too, 'OK, I'll have one last trip to the loo. Just to make sure that there's no more blood. And then that will be it. I'll just chill out and enjoy the evening.' I retraced my steps to the toilet, locked myself into the cubicle that I had vacated just minutes previously and my heart plummeted. Still fresh, still bright, still red and still, most definitely, blood. And quite a bit more of it by that point, too. And so it seemed like we didn't really have any other option. Paul and I left the pub just as our starters were being brought to the table.

... The End

We sped off to the A&E department of the hospital in the nearest, fairly small, town. I thanked my lucky stars that we had set off while Paul was still OK to drive. I had started to shiver, with the shock I suppose because I was far from cold. And so I wasn't entirely convinced that I would have been able to get us to the hospital in one piece, no matter how close by it was. At the reception desk, we gave our names and explained our situation and then, obediently, we took our seats in the waiting room.

It was Saturday night and, although it was by no means late, the place was already starting to fill up with a motley assortment of people representing various stages of inebriation. There was a happy old drunk who kept telling anyone who would listen to him that he had just stumbled and twisted his ankle and that all that he needed was a painkiller and a bandage and then he would be on his way. To the nearest pub, I had no doubt for just a drop or two more of his preferred brand of liquid painkiller. And then there were the not so happy drunks, a seemingly disproportionate number of them. And, judging by the horrendous facial injuries that they all seemed to be so proudly sporting, clearly not the type of people with whom you could make eye contact, not without a violent scuffle.

'Do you think they'll let us wait somewhere else? Somewhere more private? I think there's quite a bit more blood now. And it feels as though it's soaked through my jeans. On to the seat.'

Paul had a quiet word with the receptionist who, thankfully, was instantly sympathetic to our plight. She managed to find an unoccupied examination room for us. We hadn't moved any further up the priority list but at least we could wait our turn in privacy. And we didn't have to spend a moment longer in that horrendous waiting room.

'*Is* there blood on my jeans?' I whispered to Paul as I stood up to leave the waiting room. He handed me his jacket, to tie round my waist. I didn't look down at the seat.

Very quickly, Paul and I lost all track of time. Neither of us had been wearing watches and, because we were in a hospital, we had had to switch off our mobile phones, our only other means of telling the time. It felt as though time had all but stopped. We had nothing with which to distract ourselves, nothing even to talk about. The topic of the hour – that there was a very real chance that I was going to lose our baby – was one that just seemed too painful to voice. Neither of us was prepared to say those words out loud. Not at that stage. Not just yet.

By the time the doctor examined me, which felt like hours later, I was bleeding quite heavily. And I had started to feel very scared. I wasn't scared for myself – it was never about me. I just had this sense of almost inevitability, that this was the beginning of the end, that I was going to lose our baby and that nobody – not me, not Paul, and certainly not the overworked and under-resourced doctor who was examining me – could do a single thing about it.

I remember the doctor talking to us, talking and talking. But he kept referring to my baby, to our baby, as 'the product of conception'. And then I started crying, so I couldn't hear what he was saying any more. It was a baby to me. Not a product of conception. A baby. And I was absolutely devastated – I was heartbroken – to think that I was going to lose my baby. The doctor stopped talking, eventually, and left the room. And then a nurse came in and asked me why I was crying. And I wanted to scream at her, 'Why do you fucking think?'

I think it was just hospital procedure or local health authority procedure or some sort of procedure. But the whole experience had started to feel really quite dramatic when I was transferred to a different hospital by ambulance – to a bigger hospital, to one with a maternity ward. And what a contrast the atmosphere of that maternity ward was compared to the frantic and hassled environment of the A&E ward that we had just left. Very quickly, I felt enveloped in warmth and calmness and serenity. It was getting late. It was practically the middle of the night. The lighting in the corridors was dimmed – sleep inducingly – and it was so quiet. I could only imagine that all of the other patients were already tucked up in their hospital beds. Maybe with brand new, safely delivered babies sleeping peacefully by their sides.

I was examined for a second time. My cervix was still closed and that was a good sign, apparently. And the bleeding had slowed – it had all but stopped. And a pregnancy test said that I still was – pregnant. I allowed myself to breathe a very cautious sigh of relief. I allowed myself to hope. That maybe we were over the worst. That maybe it had just been a scare. The nurse said that I should stay in hospital overnight, anyway. Just to be on the safe side. She said that I should try to get a good night's sleep, before the hour's drive back to my parents' house. And it seemed that luck was on our side. There was a private room available, complete with an extremely welcoming looking bed. There was a reclining chair in the room, too, so Paul could stay with me. I climbed into bed and made myself comfortable. Paul settled himself into the chair beside me. And, holding hands, we slept like the safe and warm and contented babies of both of our dreams.

There was an awful lot of waiting around the next day. I needed to be examined again before I could be discharged, before I could go home. I was fairly optimistic, though. I think Paul and I both were. Overnight there hadn't been any real changes, nothing dramatic anyway. There had been a little bit of blood but nothing to get excited about. And I certainly hadn't been in any pain. The nurse who had admitted us had told us that we needed to let someone know, immediately, if things got painful. It seemed that pain could signal an ectopic pregnancy, a condition where the baby develops outside the womb, quite often in one of the fallopian tubes, a condition that could have damaging and devastating consequences on future fertility. But nothing *had* happened overnight. No pain. Nothing. And so we waited.

Paul went outside and made a few phone calls, to our parents, to a couple of friends. Just to let them know what was happening. Just to let them know where we were. And then we read magazines. We watched TV. We ate. We dozed. And we waited. Eventually, a doctor examined me. He asked me if I was feeling better and if I was in any pain and if the bleeding had abated at all and if I felt well enough to go home. Yes. No. Yes. Yes. And so, by mid-afternoon, I was finally allowed to get up. I was finally allowed to get myself ready to leave, to go home.

I decided to head to the toilet first, to change into a fresh pair of ultra glamorous, one size fits all, hospital issue paper knickers for the journey home. Home. I really could not wait to be there. And, as I sat there on the loo, my mind drifted pleasantly toward thoughts of what was waiting for me when I got home – a long soak in a nice warm bath, a clean set of clothes to change into, a mum-cooked Sunday roast with all the trimmings. And then the pleasant thoughts evaporated and my world stopped turning. I felt a sort of hot, slippery rush, like nothing I had ever experienced before. I leapt up and stared uncomprehendingly down into the toilet. And then I forced my eyes to focus on what they didn't want to see and my brain to register what it didn't want to know. The tiny beginnings of the baby that I had hoped for and dreamed about and prayed for over the last three years were lying there in that hospital toilet. The dream was over.

Numbly, I pressed the buzzer to call for the duty nurse. And the duty nurse arrived, a matter of moments later, but she was a far grumpier person than the angel who had taken such good care of Paul and me the previous night.

'Didn't they tell you last night? You're supposed to use a bedpan when you go to the loo.'

I was speechless, totally lost for words. I had just had a miscarriage – a *miscarriage* – and I was being upbraided for a minor breach of hospital ward protocol.

'I'm going to have to get that now.' She peered, with quite obvious distaste, into the toilet bowl.

I snapped back, 'Tell you what, it was my baby, I'll get it.'

The nurse backtracked – shocked, I think, by the harsh delivery of my words – and fished down into the loo. She managed to muster the sensitivity to turn her shoulder slightly, in an attempt to block what she was doing from my view, and transferred 'the product of my conception' into one of the disposable cardboard bedpans. My baby. Gone forever. I made my way back to our private room, back to Paul. And together we sobbed for lost opportunities, for unfulfilled dreams and for the loss of our much wanted and much loved baby.

Going through the Motions

We arrived home and, with an almost unbearable sense of sadness, we broke the news to my devastated parents. I had that long soak in the bath that I had promised myself. I changed into some clean clothes. I even ate a meal. And then I surprised myself. I slept soundly and dreamlessly until Monday lunchtime.

A follow up appointment had been made for me, at the hospital in the city where my parents lived. I needed to have some blood tests. To make sure that the miscarriage had been complete. That every last trace of my baby was gone. I turned up for my appointment but I didn't need the results of the blood tests to tell me what I already knew. My baby *was* gone. Every last trace of it.

I was absolutely overwhelmed by grief at first. I was heartbroken. I felt totally out of synch with the rest of the world, as though I was in some sort of no-man's-land of desolation – of emptiness – just barely able to go through the motions of my own existence. I ate, I slept and, somehow, I carried on breathing. I communicated cursorily using text messages. I couldn't face speaking to people on the phone, not even to my closest friends. And I certainly didn't want to see anyone. I didn't even want to leave the house. Paul phoned my boss, told him that I wouldn't be back at work for at least a week. Maybe more. I cried off from a friend's baby's christening. I think that they understood. I hope that they did. And, very gradually, my tears became less and less ready. We began to make some tentative arrangements for the future, Paul and me, to revisit some of our plans and to make some decisions. And we relied on the strength of our relationship to give us courage and to give us hope.

Plan A

I had never been a particularly great believer in fate. I always used to think that what you got out of life was in direct proportion to what you put in. That success was more about how hard you worked than the cards that life had dealt you. I thought that you created your own opportunities in life, plain and simple. But two things – fate, luck, coincidence, chance, serendipity, call them what you will – happened during that first month after my miscarriage that made me change my mind.

Unanimously, Paul and I had made the decision to revert back to Plan A. We *would* leave our jobs, leave my family, leave our friends and start a new life for ourselves in Ireland. I handed in my notice at work and my boss duly issued a note to the business, to our customers, to our suppliers. To let them know that I was relocating to Ireland, to let them know when I would be leaving, and let them know who would be replacing me. During the four and a half years that I had been at the company, my phone and my email inbox had never seen such action. Colleagues wanting an inside-track on the gossip behind my resignation story. Others wanting to wish me well. And one of the company's suppliers, calling to make me an offer that I couldn't refuse.

I had worked with the same packaging design agency for years, for so long, in fact, that they had started to feel more like colleagues than suppliers. And, as it turned out – luckily, coincidentally, fatefully – the timing of my relocation to Ireland fitted perfectly with their plans for expansion into new markets, into Irish markets. It looked as though, without even trying, I had got myself lined up with some freelance marketing work.

And then, one day, my dad gave me a ring at work. He had been talking to one of my cousins and he had told her that Paul and I were planning to move to Ireland just as soon as I had worked out my notice. And, almost incredibly, it turned out that one of my cousin's friends had a holiday home close to the small Kerry town that Paul and I had fallen in love with in the summer. And, luckily, coincidentally, fatefully – my cousin's friend knew a woman with a house to rent. A house that was newly built, a house that was reasonably priced, a house that was available immediately. And so it looked as though, without even trying, Paul and I had got ourselves a place to live too.

Opinions Are like Ass-holes, Everyone Has One

Since the other elements of our new life seemed to have fallen so very neatly into place – we had got a plan, I had got myself a job, we had got ourselves a place to live – that first month after my miscarriage, I felt incredibly frustrated, almost ungratefully so and certainly unrealistically so, that I hadn't immediately found myself pregnant again. I was frustrated that the final piece of the jigsaw, the one that really would have made the picture of our life complete, should so stubbornly continue to refuse to fall into position.

I knew that it was extremely unlikely for me to conceive that first month after my miscarriage. And, at first, I almost managed to convince myself that I wasn't even trying to conceive again. I almost managed to convince myself that I was concentrating on getting my body back to normal first, that I was concentrating on letting my hormones settle themselves down. But then I ovulated on exactly the day that I thought I would. And the timing of our first post-miscarriage sex couldn't have been any better if we *had* planned it. And then I realized that I hadn't suffered from my usual array of PMT symptoms either. No moodiness. No uncontrollable urges to spring clean. No spottiness. No carbohydrate cravings. Just tiredness.

Extreme, immobilizing tiredness. And I tried really hard, at first, to stop my mind from going down the 'that's exactly how you felt when you were pregnant' route. But then I just gave in. I let myself get swept away by the maybes. The slightest little thing became a symptom, a sign, almost a surety. Until, by the end of it all, I was totally and thoroughly convinced that I was, indeed, pregnant. I even did a pregnancy test; quite sure the result would simply confirm what I already knew. But it didn't. All that it did was prove me wrong. I failed the pregnancy test miserably, in more ways than one.

A friend once told me that she felt like she had become public property as soon as she had got pregnant, as soon as she had a visible bump. And, in the months after my miscarriage, I knew exactly how she felt. Only without the baby bump. (Unless, of course, I was indulging in the old pillow-up-the-jumper, imagining-I-was-pregnant routine. But I was still managing to keep that particular little charade to myself, confined to the privacy of my own bedroom ...) I felt as though the world and his dog knew what Paul and I were going through. Family, friends, colleagues and neighbours – it seemed as though everyone had an opinion and an opinion that they felt duty bound to share with us.

'Well at least you know that you can get pregnant now.' Yes. How reassuring it was to know that after more than three years of trying for a baby, I could at least get pregnant enough to have a miscarriage. Hmm.

'Quite often a miscarriage is a sign that something was wrong with the baby, you know.' OK. After more than three years of trying for a baby, at least I could get pregnant enough to miscarry an abnormal one – even more reassuring.

'Loads of my other friends have had miscarriages. They were all pregnant again within six months.' Great. So the clock was ticking and the pressure was on. I had to make sure that I got pregnant again before the year was out.

'Do you know what? You just need to keep nice and relaxed about it all.' How, God help me, how?

Plenty of Questions, Just Not Enough Answers

Years ago – long before the experience had affected me personally, long before it had started to colour almost every aspect of my life – I remember reading somewhere that infertility was one of the most emotionally difficult life situations that one could ever have to deal with. That it was worse than dealing with a terminal illness or worse than dealing with the aftermath of a serious accident. That it was worse, even, than dealing with the death of someone close. And I remember disagreeing at the time. I remember dismissing the very notion as over dramatic, as sensationalistic even. But then I reached a stage in our own experience of infertility when I could see that whoever had written that had hit the nail firmly on the head.

My own extremely painful experience of involuntary childlessness seemed to call into question some of the most basic – some of the most *fundamental* – expectations that I had about myself, about my relationship with Paul, about my future and about my life. And, of course, there were no easy answers to the deep and philosophical questions that infertility had raised for me. Who was I – what was I – if I was never going to become a mother? And was it really possible to miss something that you had never even had?

Who Am I, if I'm Never Going to Become a Mother?

Whenever I had thought about the future, the future that was waiting for Paul and me, it had always been a case of 'when we have children' rather than 'if we have children'. That future family of ours had always seemed to be so tangible and real, it had always seemed to be just around the corner. And, maybe naively, I had assumed that when the time was right for me – when the time was right for *us* – the baby thing would just happen. But when the baby thing *didn't* just happen, month after month, it started to feel as though all of my expectations about life were slowly but surely being turned on their heads. As the months passed, I realized that I needed to rethink almost everything that I had previously taken for granted. I had to rethink my expectations about conception and pregnancy, about childbirth and babies, about children and family life. I had to rethink my expectations about our marriage and about our life, in general. I had to rethink almost everything that I had taken for granted about our future. Because everything that I had taken for granted about our future, everything that I had been moving toward, everything that I had been *working* toward seemed destined to remain out of reach.

I had always imagined that raising a family would be my major preoccupation throughout my thirties and forties. And, I remember wondering, if that wasn't going to be the case, then what was? All of the beliefs that I had held about things like employment, about financial security, about property ownership and even about things like savings plans suddenly seemed largely redundant. If there was only ever going to be me and Paul to worry about, then what did it matter if we spent our last days in some rented shack, penniless or even up to our ears in debt?

Also, I had got so used to other people telling Paul and me that we would be great parents. I had got so used to other people telling Paul and me that we would be *perfect* parents. It was hard for me to get my head around the fact that Paul and I might never be parents at all, great or perfect or otherwise. That Paul and I might well have to resign ourselves to a future of childlessness. *Childlessness.* Just the word alone was enough to strike a cold sense of dread into my heart. It was just so bleak sounding and so hopeless and so negative.

I tried to imagine myself as being childless, as being permanently childless. And I imagined myself as a middle-aged woman, grey and colourless and dry and staid. I imagined myself with a houseful of cats, cats that were the sole recipients of an abundance of maternal love that, clearly, wasn't required elsewhere, cats that were the sole recipients of an abundance of maternal love that would otherwise have gone to waste because I really didn't know what else to do with it. And I felt as though I just couldn't bear it.

When I thought about childless women, I thought about frustrated and embittered ones. I thought about hard-bitten corporate high-flyers. I thought about ball-breaking men-haters. I thought about the baddies in films, about characters like Cruella de Vil, about women like Myra Hindley. And so I suppose it was hardly surprising that I didn't feel in any particular hurry to sign myself up to the childless woman's Hall of Fame.

But as the months and the years went by – and Paul and I continued to try for our baby without success – the more difficult it became for me to ever picture myself being a mother. And so I found it increasingly hard to even *attempt* to empathize with the growing legion of pregnant women and new mothers that seemed to be surrounding me. Their gripes about morning sickness and weight gain, about swollen ankles and the pain of labour, about stretch marks and sleepless nights, about the cost of nappies and the paucity of decent child care, about the loss of freedom and of spontaneity, all seemed to me such a very small price to pay for the incredible gift of having a child of your own.

But, no matter how I was feeling inside, I would bite my lip. I would hold my tongue. I would try my absolute best to just grin and bear it. I would nod and make the appropriate noises when women told me about how awful it was for them, getting pregnant and having babies. What else could I have done?

Most of my friends, and certainly all of my close friends, either had kids or planned to have them. I remember, at one particularly painful time for me, the grand total of five of my friends being pregnant – and, since I wasn't prepared to lose contact with all of the women of child-bearing age in my address book, I really didn't feel as though I had an awful lot of choice.

Can You Miss What You Have Never Had?

Because our infertility was unexplained infertility, and because I *had* managed to get pregnant before, there was always a chance that one day I would conceive again, naturally and spontaneously. And so it was almost impossible to know when to say that enough was enough. It was almost impossible to know when to say that Paul and I were no longer trying for a baby; that we were just going to get on with the rest of our life. And although I found it incredibly hard – staying positive, keeping going, carrying on *trying* – I didn't know when was the right time to let myself get realistic either. I didn't know when was the right time to let myself start grieving, about our not having had a child.

Our experience of unexplained infertility meant that I never really felt as though Paul and I had reached the end of the road. Not quite. It always seemed as though there was a glimmer of hope – no matter how faint, no matter how small – a new drug to try, a new treatment of some sort, a different alternative therapy. And so what could I do? Postpone my sadness until I had exhausted every last possible type of medical treatment and every last possible remedy and every last possible technique? Or did I have to wait even longer than that before I could finally let myself mourn for my involuntary childlessness, mourn for my sense of loss? Did I have to wait until I had reached the menopause, until there really was absolutely no chance of my ever getting pregnant again?

And I found it so difficult to put into words, even to myself, the full extent of my sadness – a sadness that seemed so fundamental and yet, at the same time, so intangible. Was my sadness about the ghosts of my children who would never actually be born? Was it about missing out on the reputedly life-enhancing experience of pregnancy, of childbirth, of motherhood? Was it about never having the opportunity to read bedtime stories to my own children, to tuck them in, to kiss them goodnight, to tell them how much I loved them? Was it about never hearing someone exclaim, 'My God! She's the image of you'? Was it about feeling as though I was a failure as a woman – socially and biologically and genetically and personally? Was it about being unable to carry out what seemed – for other women – to be a fairly basic and straightforward human function?

I read an absolutely fascinating book once. In it, women were asked to list all of the reasons why they wanted to have a baby, why they wanted to have a family. And their responses certainly made for interesting reading. Some women said that they wanted to have a baby so that they could feel feminine, so that they could feel fulfilled as a woman and as a human being. Some women said that they wanted to have a baby to feel as though they had *made* something with their partners, so that they could pass on their genes, so that they could have someone to remember them after they had gone. Some said that they wanted to have a baby so that they could enjoy the status of being a mother, so that they could have a clearly defined role, so that they could have a purpose in life. Some said that they wanted to have a baby so that they could give love and receive it. And some women said that they wanted to have a baby so that they could be just like everybody else. And, to be honest, I felt as though I knew where every single one of those women was coming from.

And a lot of the time, I found it incredibly confusing, *not* having a baby. A lot of the time, I didn't really know what to think. I didn't really know what to *feel*. It wasn't as though somebody had died – not some living, once-breathing person with a birth certificate to prove that they had been real, to prove that they had existed. But, looking back, with the benefit of hindsight I think I did need to mourn just as though somebody had died. Because I felt somebody or some*thing* had. I needed to grieve for my unborn children, but I really didn't have a clue where to begin. I am pretty sure that I would have benefited from a few sessions with a bereavement counsellor. Maybe some counselling would have been good for both of us – for Paul *and* me – to help us to acknowledge our very real sense of loss and to work through it and to move on from it. But I decided to take up yoga instead, to help me to get my head together. And Paul and I decided to look toward the future and to start getting excited about our new life together in Ireland.

Learning to Breathe

I found myself a twice-weekly yoga class, just around the corner from my mum and dad's house. I had always fancied taking up yoga properly – I had bought myself a couple of DVDs, years before, trying to teach myself the basics at home – and I resisted the urge to put it off until we moved to Ireland. I didn't want Ireland to become this mythical place, where everything would be different, where everything would be OK, where our new and improved life could start. Paul and I were planning to be in England for another two months and I didn't want to waste that time. I remember being keen for my new and improved life to start there and then.

It was amazing, my first yoga class. I felt as though I had become properly aware of my body for the first time in my life. I remember shrugging my shoulders toward my ears and then letting them drop back down with a sigh. I felt as though I was shrugging off years of anxiety and tension and frustration. And when we moved on to the breathing exercises – where we practised the deep and nourishing breathing techniques that our bodies really need – I felt as though I had been holding my breath for most of my adult life. As the heady mix of oxygen and relaxation coursed through my body, I felt incredibly moved, close to tears, in fact, when I realized just how tense I had been for so very long.

Yoga just ticked so many boxes for me, on so many different levels. It was a great form of exercise, for a start. After my first couple of classes I felt trimmer and leaner. I felt longer and more supple. My posture seemed better and I started to feel much more positive about myself and about my body. During those yoga classes, I felt as though my body was doing something natural, as though it was doing something good. As though I was living and breathing and being. I wasn't hunched over my computer or trapped in my car in yet another traffic jam or caught up in the twenty-first century's obsession with doing, doing, doing. I had a couple of hours a week that were just for me, that were for peace and for reflection – an escape from the rest of the world. And I felt as though I was gradually resuming control of my body and my health and my life. While Paul and I had been trying (and failing) to have a baby, I had started to feel let down by my body. While Paul and I had been undergoing fertility treatment, I felt as though I had just handed over the responsibility for my body and for my health and for my fertility to the medical professionals. But yoga helped me to feel ready to take back that responsibility.

After my yoga classes, I invariably felt light and positive. I felt hopeful and creative. I invariably felt as though I was looking forward to meeting life's problems and challenges rather than feeling overwhelmed by them. And, as the weeks passed, I became seduced by the whole concept of 'me-time', by the whole concept of time dedicated to relaxation. And then I spotted an advert for a reflexology practitioner and I decided to get myself another piece of the in-action.

Walking On Air

The quite significant holes in my knowledge about reflexology as an alternative therapy were appropriately filled when I called to make my first appointment. I found out that the underlying principle of reflexology was that different areas or zones within both the hands and the feet correspond to every single organ and system within the body from the kidneys to the respiratory system. I found out that by manipulating these different areas, usually in the feet, physical problems in the corresponding areas of the body – caused by illness or by toxins or even by stress – could be alleviated. And that not only could reflexology help to restore equilibrium to the mind and the body by returning energy flow to a fully functioning and natural state, but it was also incredibly relaxing, too. And so that was it. I was completely sold on the idea of reflexology.

The first fifteen minutes of my first reflexology session were basically a knowledge exchange. I found out about what to expect during my treatment (a touch of discomfort, possibly, as energy blockages were discovered and removed) and what to expect after my treatment (sleep, sleep and more sleep, apparently). And the reflexologist found out about my diet (on the whole healthy with the occasional sinful indulgence) and about my lifestyle (ditto). And then she asked me if I was experiencing any particular health problems.

I demurred from telling her at first, my inner cynic goading, 'Oh come on. If reflexology is as good as it's cracked up to be, she'll be able to tell what's wrong with you as soon as she gets your socks off.' But then I decided to spill the beans anyway. And so I told her all about my emotionally and physically draining experience of infertility and about my miscarriage and about my fears that I would never get pregnant again, my fears that I would never have children. And I luxuriated in the experience of being able to just talk – about me, myself, and I – without having to brace myself for the usually inevitable, 'You know what I would do …' And, when I came up for air, I felt such a sense of lightness, such a sense of unburdening that that alone would have been worth the price of the session.

But the treatment was amazing. Small hot spots of tension just seemed to melt away under the therapist's fingers. And the words of my inner cynic melted away with them. I was amazed when the reflexologist asked me if I was having any problems with my teeth. Because, just the day before, I had noticed that a filling in one of my back teeth felt a little bit wobbly. And I thought that the filling probably needed to be replaced. And so I had made a note for myself in my diary, a reminder to give my dentist a call, to see about getting the filling replaced before Paul and I left for Ireland. I was astounded that the reflexologist had been able to pick up on the problem – such a minor one – just from working on my feet. She pinpointed areas of tension in my shoulders, too. And she noticed that I was dehydrated; she told me that I needed to make a conscious effort to drink lots more water in order to help flush toxins from my system.

When I eventually stood up to leave almost an hour later, I felt weightless, as though I was floating several inches above the ground, as though I was walking on air. I felt refreshed and revitalized; as though I'd just woken from a particularly deep sleep, as though I'd just drunk a long, cool glass of water, or a weight had been lifted from my shoulders. And I decided to put my name down for a reflexology session every week until Paul and I left for Ireland.

Running, Just as Fast as We Can?

⌣⟶

I had mixed feelings, in the last few weeks before we moved to Ireland. I was excited, first and foremost. There was something incredibly appealing about being able to have a completely fresh start in life – the clean slate of a brand new life in a brand new country, where Paul and I could both be whatever we wanted to be. Where our dreams could come true. And both of us had so many dreams, we both had so many plans.

Paul had had a great idea for a business – helping people to sell their homes without using an estate agent. And since we were going to be renting a place to live, for our first year in Ireland at least, without the pressure of mortgage repayments, we were pretty hopeful about Paul's chances of getting his business idea off the ground. I was going to do the freelance marketing work that I had been offered, just for a couple of days a week, just to earn enough money to cover the bills. And I was going to write. Finally. After dreaming about it since childhood. I was going to try my hand at writing for a living. Paul and I both had lots of things to look forward to.

But moving away did feel as though it was the end of something, too, as though it was the end of an era. Certain aspects of our life in England had already changed fairly dramatically.

Our social life, for a start, had become a shadow of its former self. Paul and I used to be out and about pretty much every weekend – for anything from informally impromptu get-togethers with a handful of friends to full on social events that had been months in the planning. But gradually, as more and more kids had come along, our friends had started to need three months' advance warning before they would even leave the house. And previously reliably up-for-it mates would drop out at a moment's notice because one of their children had sneezed. When I thought about it, I missed my friends already. Even though I still lived in the same country, in the same county and in some cases even in the same town, I missed them.

And so maybe there was a certain sense of running away, too. Running away from a way of life that seemed to be a constant reminder of our failure to have children, from the friends who seemed to be popping babies out by the dozen. Running away from a society that presented life as a series of boxes to be ticked: education, career, husband, mortgage, children – and, ideally, in that order. And from a media that represented parenthood, albeit a sugar-coated and idealized version of parenthood, as the pinnacle of human achievement.

'Every time I turn on the TV, there's some rosy cheeked family happily – lovingly – taking turns to open their presents or tucking into a perfectly roasted turkey with all of the trimmings or pulling crackers and laughing. It's enough to make you throw up. Or slit your wrists.' There I was, immersing myself fully into the Christmas spirit.

'Believe it or not ...' My friend had three adorable children so, at first, I was more inclined to 'not'. '... I feel exactly the same way that you do. Nobody's Christmas is like that. There's always someone crying because their Barbie princess isn't quite as magical as she appeared in the TV ad or someone spitting out their sprouts or screaming, terrified by the noise of the crackers. My experience of the perfect family Christmas – even with the kids – is as far from ideal as yours is.'

And I remember thinking that, when we moved to Ireland, Paul and I could redefine our Christmases. We could turn them into something more meaningful for ourselves.

She's Leaving Home

Our last week in England was like being transported back to our social whirl of old. Paul and I were out every single night of that week kissing goodbye to our colleagues and to our friends and to my family. And I remember thinking what a shame it was – what a *waste* it was – that all of us seemed to have to wait for an event, like a leaving party, before we could pluck up the courage to tell those closest to us how we really feel about them. Before we can tell them that we love them, that we will miss them, that our lives will be a little bit emptier without them. Without such a catalyst, it seems it can be all too easy to take people for granted. To assume that your family and your friends, all of the people you really care about, will always be there and so you have all the time in the world to tell them what they mean to you. And so you can wait indefinitely – until the next week or the next month, until the next year or the next decade. You can wait forever.

I didn't realize, until that week of goodbyes, just how many people I was going to miss or just how many people were going to miss me. Maybe it was just as well. Perhaps Paul and I never would have gone, if we had known. But it was too late. We had booked our ferry tickets – one way – and we had packed our bags and we had shoehorned our possessions – cat included – into the car. And so that was it. We were going to Ireland.

Caed Mile Failte

It was like being on holiday at first. Our rented house was in an amazingly picturesque location, halfway up a mountain with stunning uninterrupted views of fields and rivers, of forests and hills. When I opened the curtains in the morning, I would stare out through the window for ages, mesmerized by the picture postcard beauty of it all. And it was just so peaceful. The occasional forestry lorry would pass, loaded with logs. We would hear bird song a sheep or a cow or a donkey would break the silence, sporadically. But that was pretty much it.

The silence and the stillness and the inky darkness at night – the nearest street light was half an hour's drive away, along with the 'local' shop – took a little bit of getting used to, for both of us. Before we moved to Ireland, I had heard the expression that silence could be deafening but I had never really understood what it meant. But during our first few nights in Ireland, when the silence kept me awake – no late buses or car alarms, no drunken neighbours or HGVs – I slowly began to understand.

We gave ourselves a little bit of time to settle in, to explore the local area and to find the best places to take visiting friends and family. We found the best places for freshly caught seafood and for typical Irish fare; for a long walk on a deserted beach and for a day of horse racing; for a night on the Guinness and for the best chance of catching an impromptu traditional music session; for strolls to spectacular waterfalls and through forest parks and to castles; for locally made glass and cheese and pottery and chocolate. And we spent some time getting to know our new neighbours, too.

Our next-door neighbours were the absolute epitome of Irish hospitality. I don't think that it would have been humanly possible for our neighbours to make us feel any more welcome than they did. 'You'll come in for a cup of tea?' A rhetorical question as we arrived after a long drive on our first day in Ireland – to collect the keys for our new home. And, very quickly, I began to realize that in certain parts of Ireland 'a cup of tea' was a euphemism for a bottomless pot of tea and a tray full of ham sandwiches, a homemade cake and a tin of biscuits, a good long chat in front of a roaring fire and a drop or two of 'mountain dew'. And so it was getting late by the time we headed next door – to our new house – but our neighbours still insisted on helping us to unload our car. And then they handed us another bag to unpack, a brown paper bag full of bread and butter and ham and cheese and milk and tea and a fresh apple tart. And I remember getting a very good feeling about our move.

Breathing out and Letting Go

Gradually, I felt as though I was starting to unwind, as though I was actually starting to relax and for days and days at a time – not just for the couple of hours a week that I had allocated to the job of relaxation when we were living in England, not just during a yoga class or during a reflexology session. And I realized just how stressed out I had been before. Stressed by the sense that I was drifting away from my friends, feeling out of touch with them, especially the ones with kids, as though we were losing our common ground. Stressed by the feeling that our spontaneous and affectionate lovemaking had turned into diarized and pressurized baby making and – as if that wasn't bad enough – that it wasn't working. Stressed by the gradual replacement of passion and tenderness with resentment and bitterness. By inconclusive test findings and failed fertility treatments. By the sense of loss and feelings of despair and hopelessness that I had experienced after my miscarriage. By feeling out of control of my fertility and my health and my body and even my future. I am not exactly sure how depression is defined but I think that I was probably getting pretty close to it at one stage. I think that Paul and I both were.

And, from what I had read, if the anxiety and the stress, the unhappiness and the frustration don't get in there first with their negative impact on your ability to conceive then a bout of depression most definitely will. And all of the advice that I had read seemed to point in the same direction. Teach yourself some de-stressing techniques, anything that works for you, anything that helps you to relax. And, in our first few months in Ireland, Paul and I had all the time in the world to do just that.

De-stressing Techniques – Irish Style

We managed to find ourselves a couple of short courses, locally. Paul had always been interested in photography but when we had been living in England, he had just never found the time to take it up. He quickly found himself an evening class, run by a relocated Californian. And he loved it. I started a counselling course, just an introductory one – and the course helped me to get to know myself better as well as giving me a great opportunity to get up close and personal with a few of the locals. I joined a writers' group, the weekly meetings helping to give some much needed focus to my own writing. And I found myself a new yoga teacher.

I loved my weekly yoga classes and I felt an instant connection, an instant rapport, with my yoga teacher. And the two of us got chatting one day, after a class, over a pot of herbal tea. My yoga teacher told me that she wanted to create some awareness about her approach to yoga and about her yoga centre. She told me that she would really like to do some marketing but that she didn't know where to begin. And I told her that I would love to have private yoga tuition but that, with no regular income, I didn't really feel as though I could justify the cost. And then we looked at each other and we laughed, because the ideal basis for a bartering arrangement was staring both of us in the face. An hour's worth of marketing for an hour's worth of yoga. Perfect.

I started to exercise most days. Going to classes or to my personal yoga tuition. Chasing sheep back up on to the mountain or bringing donkeys back down from it. Having a good long walk – and in the middle of the day too and in the middle of the week – it gave my strolls a delicious sense of truancy. And I managed to find the time to really pamper myself. There had never seemed to be much time for pampering when Paul and I had been living in England. Pampering had been a rare sort of treat – an hour or so at the hairdresser's a couple of times a year, my annual pilgrimage to a spa with a group of friends. And I would always be full of good intentions, after my spa trip, determined that I was going to maintain *some* sort of beauty routine when I got home. And my good intentions would last for a couple of weeks at the most before taking the time to indulge myself, to *beautify* myself, slipped right off the bottom of my priority list. But, in Ireland, all of that changed. I invested in a bathroom cabinet's worth of beauty goodies. I bought manicure kits and home facials. I bought hair conditioning packs and fake tan. And I had never felt so buffed and so polished. I had never felt so *tanned*. Thinking about one particularly successful in-home tanning session, one that I had done just before going home for a family wedding, because I had wanted to go back to England looking fit and healthy, still makes me chuckle. My tanning session had been so successful that my freshly bronzed appearance had taken one of our neighbours by surprise.

'Do you know, Isla, I hardly recognized you!' he had exclaimed, only half-joking. And then he had quipped, 'Now, will everyone in England not be wanting to move to Ireland? When they see what gorgeous, tropical weather we've been having?'

Becoming Local

The weather wasn't *particularly* tropical on our first St Patrick's Day in Ireland but it was beautiful and bright, it was fresh and spring-like. And so Paul and I decided to head out for the day. We headed out to our local small town to watch the St Patrick's Day parade. And we giggled at the floats – mainly hordes of children, crammed on to the back of trailers, smiling and waving at the crowds, wearing costumes that were impossible to distinguish – although I'm still not a hundred per cent sure that they were meant to be funny. And then we took the scenic route home. Actually we *inched* our way along the scenic route home with Paul pulling over at regular intervals after spotting 'great photo opportunities' and evidently great photo opportunities that really couldn't be missed. And as the hours passed, our festive liquid dinner at the local pub called – somehow an alcohol embargo would have just felt wrong in Ireland, on St Patrick's Day of all days.

Festive liquid dinners aside, our life in Ireland quickly started to revolve around food. From the home baked scones and crusty brown bread and freshly caught fish that our neighbours brought round for us, to a steak house close by with such locally supplied meat that you could practically work out which cow you were eating by looking out of the window and seeing which one was missing from the field, Paul and I soon got to know the ways of the countryside. And I quickly found myself on first name terms with our next-door neighbours' donkeys.

I remember spending a very different sort of morning – in borrowed and too-big wellies – trying to catch a couple of them. Jack and Oisin (the donkeys, not the neighbours) had escaped out of their field and up on to the mountain at the back of our house. One of our neighbours had asked me if I would help her to try and catch them. Catching them was the easy part. Trying to persuade the donkeys to come back down the mountain with us was a very different story. Stubborn as a mule – I had never quite appreciated the aptness of the description before.

'Help me!' I squeaked, as Jack, the donkey, had edged closer and closer toward me, eyeballing me, unblinkingly, the whole time.

'Oh he's just being friendly.' Somehow the idea of a 'friendly' donkey with a glint of mischief in his eyes wasn't particularly reassuring.

Another donkey, Rosie, had clearly already been on the receiving end of Jack's particular brand of friendliness. And she gave birth to a tiny foal during our first summer in Ireland. As gorgeous – all wobbly legged and long eye-lashed and fluffy coated – as only a baby donkey can be. And Paul and I were asked to celebrate the new arrival with our neighbours. We celebrated with hot toddies, heavy on the whisky. And I was delighted and felt incredibly honoured to be asked to choose her name. I still blame the whisky drinking – unaccustomed – at any time of the day, never mind at half past eleven in the morning – for my somewhat uninspired choice. Daisy.

As our first few months in Ireland passed, I noticed that the contents of my wardrobe gradually evolved. They had gone from the impossibly impractical – and subsequently ruined – embroidered turquoise silk flip-flops that I had decided to wear down to a local sheep shearing event, to garments and footwear of a much more comfortable and warm – and quite uncharacteristically for me – practical nature. And, as our first few months in Ireland passed, Paul and I started to think about putting down some roots.

We started to give some thought to building a house of our own from scratch and we talked to a neighbour about how to go about getting hold of a decent piece of land for ourselves. And then we started to sketch out some ideas. Paul's ideas were all very grand designs – all glass floors and galleries and split level living. My house ideas were a bit more grounded in practicality – and much more limited by drawing ability. I included things like storage space – thinking that you can never have too much – and an outside utility area for bins and compost heaps and a washing line and a shed. And I found myself becoming something of a house layout anorak. I would spend hours, thinking about all of the houses that I had ever been in, sketching out their room arrangements and scoring them for a) convenience and b) aesthetic appeal. But what the hell, it certainly helped me to take my mind off *not* having a baby.

Mind, Body and Spirit

During our first few months in Ireland, I had managed to shake off the sense of desperation that I had started to feel whenever I thought about pregnancy and babies and families. I still wanted to have a baby. Paul and I *both* still wanted to have a baby. But there were so many other things happening in our life that 'the baby thing' could no longer occupy every waking hour. I was taking better care of my general health and well-being than I had done in years and I had started to feel as though I was really in touch with my body and mind again. I started to feel much more aware of my physical and emotional needs and our newly flexible lifestyle meant that not only did I have the time to really *listen* to what my body was telling me but that I could respond to it too.

I ate when I was hungry rather than just grabbing something when it was convenient. And I slept when I was tired. I didn't have to force myself to try and get to sleep at ten o'clock any more, there wasn't any rush hour traffic to contend with and so I didn't have to get up again at six. And I started to meditate, too. I taught myself a very simple technique – just sitting comfortably and quietly and letting myself become aware of my breath. And the great thing was that I could use it anywhere, whenever I needed to. I carried on listening to my

Hypnotherapy for Fertility CD. And I really did feel as though I was soothing away all the negative messages that I had stored, unconsciously, about pregnancy and childbirth and motherhood.

I met a local alternative therapist too. And she told me about a new type of approach that she had been learning about, an approach that might be of interest to me. It was called the Dawson Programme and it combined kinesiology and sound therapy. All of this was new information for me but the new Irish version of me, relaxed and receptive and open to new possibilities, was willing to give it a go.

I discovered that kinesiology is based on the concept that illnesses – caused by emotional issues or by disease, by dysfunction or by toxins, by nutritional deficiencies or by stress – can manifest themselves as muscle weaknesses or as postural problems. I found out that, in an ideal world, energy would be flowing freely around everyone's body and nourishing every cell and every organ. But that illnesses, no matter how minor, can cause blockages and that blocked energy isn't good energy. And so the muscles are tested, in kinesiology, to check for any weaknesses that might indicate problems in other parts of the body.

I remember feeling a bit sceptical at first, not to say just a little bit vulnerable, as I lay on my back with my arm in the air, trying to resist the downward pressure of the kinesiologist as she tested my muscles. She told me that she had, quite quickly, uncovered a well of sadness and a deep sense of unfairness. I had already told her about our struggle to have a baby so I wasn't entirely convinced, at first, that this was anything more impressive than guesswork. And then came the really strange part. Sound therapy.

The thinking behind the Dawson Programme is that problems identified during the muscle-testing bit of the treatment can be resolved using sound – or, more specifically, energy in the form of sound. I'm still not sure if I entirely understand the principle of sound therapy but the kinesiologist told me that different parts of the body vibrate at different frequencies and that by applying sound at the correct frequency the body can start to heal itself. Immediately. With no more treatment required. I still wasn't convinced but I paid for my treatment anyway and I drove myself home.

Maybe it was the placebo effect. Maybe it had done me more good than I had realized to just lie down for an hour, listening to relaxing music and to a soothing voice and to the peal of bells. Or maybe it had actually worked. When I arrived home, I realized that I felt incredibly happy and upbeat and that I was really looking forward to the future.

Time Flies ...

And yet, just a couple of months after my Dawson Programme treatment, I panicked. Any sense of calmness and well-being, happiness and hope seemed to desert me. And I had this almost overwhelming sense that time and opportunities were running out on me, that I was never going to have children and that despite all of my attempts at being philosophical and thinking positively and counting my blessings, I really was not OK with the prospect of my own childlessness. I still don't know what triggered it. It could have been something to do with the fast approaching due date for the baby that I had miscarried in the summer. It could have been the fact that my thirty-third birthday was just around the corner and with it the fourth anniversary of when Paul and I had made the decision to start trying for our baby. Or maybe I had just read one too many depressing newspaper articles about women in their mid-thirties trying, desperately, to beat the biological clock.

I had read once that if you feel young enough to have a baby then you probably are young enough to have a baby. But it was becoming increasingly difficult, for me, to find any comfort in that thought. At the forefront of my mind was the widely reported 'fact' that sixteen was the optimum age, physically, to conceive a child. And that it all went downhill, fertility-wise, after that. That once you had reached the grand old age of thirty-five, an age that all of a sudden seemed frighteningly close for me, you had pretty much had it.

My imminent birthday had started to feel as though it was something to fear rather than something to celebrate – another year older and yet another year without a baby. And my birthday had seemed to take on an almost New Year's-like quality, but not in a good way. There was all of the introspection and taking stock and comparing dreams with reality and attempting to predict the future. This time next year …' But there was none of the drunken celebration with friends.

I tried to be rational. I knew that there was no way that I would have been ready to start a family as a teenager. And I remember wondering who would be ready to have a baby at that age? How many women (or men, come to think of it) are still with the partners that they had when they were sixteen? And what about all of the other non-baby related hopes and dreams? Things like freedom and an education, some fun and a career? Did it really have to be a case of either/or?

And then I tried to tell myself that thirty-three wasn't exactly *old* – I was far from being in my dotage. But no matter how hard I tried to be rational and logical, I couldn't quite shake off the feeling that time was running out for me. I couldn't quite shake off the feeling that if I didn't do something drastic – and soon – there was going to be nothing left for me on the baby shelf.

... Whether You're Having Fun or Not

When Paul and I had made the decision to start trying for our baby, the thought of actually being pregnant, of giving birth to a baby, of raising a family was pretty hazy and shadowy for me. I did have a vague sort of notion about being proud and delighted about an impossibly neat little baby bump. But then I would skim over the gory bits and the painful bits until I was happily cuddling my very own sweet smelling, and usually sleeping child. But that dreaminess and that vagueness and that shadowiness seemed to change rather dramatically. It seemed to transform into something sharp edged and crystal clear. My desire, my need, my wish, my *want* for a child of my own became absolutely tangible. I could see it, I could hear it, I could touch it – I could almost smell it, I could almost taste it.

Having a baby began to seem, to me, to be the very pinnacle of female creativity. It seemed, to me, to be the very essence of female *purpose*. The urge to hold in my arms a child that we had created – Paul and me – became almost overwhelming. It became a *requirement*. The biological urge to procreate, to reproduce, felt like an instinct that was almost animal but at the same time, was very, very human. All of a sudden, it felt as though every cell in my body was crying out for a child.

My days and my nights – awake and asleep – were filled with vivid and emotionally charged images. I imagined the happy summers of my childhood and joyful family Christmases and birthdays filled with laughter and love. I imagined all of the things that I might never be able to experience with a child of my own. And I imagined myself as the perpetual babysitter – an amiable auntie looking after other people's children – but never as the mother figure of my dreams.

The fear that I would never have a child of my own, that I would never have a child with Paul, became absolutely tangible too. It felt incredibly real and physically painful. I began to fear that I would never know the comfort and the security of a brand new generation. It wasn't about there being nobody to look after me when I was old and frail – it wasn't about that at all. I don't think that I could even have borne to look that far ahead. It was about something much more primal than that. It was about something like it being the end of the line for Paul and me, genetically speaking. My own mortality felt infinitely more concrete without the prospect of a child that I could entrust with all the old family stories and with my personal effects and with the dubious legacy of a rather distinctive family nose. And I was really unhappy about that. I was really unhappy because it left me with a dreadful sense of finality.

Weighing up the Options

I told Paul how I was feeling and we talked it over, trying to come up with a plan, one that we were both happy with. Neither of us was prepared to go down the IVF route. I had read all that I needed to read about its phenomenally low success rates and about its horrendous side effects and about marriages breaking apart under the strain of it. I didn't want to subject myself to that – I didn't want to subject either of us to that – not until there really was absolutely no other alternative.

'I just don't feel ready to go down the IVF route … In fact, I'm not sure that I'll ever feel ready to go down the IVF route.'

'I know what you mean …'

'I just remember how badly Clomid affected me, how negatively I felt about IUI and, from what I've heard, both of those things are a walk in the park compared to IVF.'

'I know. Remember that leaflet that we picked up at the fertility clinic? *Ravaged by Baby Hunger*?'

'God, how could I forget? Talk about painting a dark picture. That poor woman lost everything – her home, her job, her relationship – and she still didn't have a baby at the end of it.'

'I suppose that's the thing with IVF though, isn't it? I suppose that's the thing with any fertility treatment. The chances are that it's *not* going to work. All treatments are much more likely to fail than they are to succeed.'

'And that's the thing that I struggle with most. That there aren't any guarantees. No one can say to you – look, just give it a go or give it three goes or five goes or whatever. And then there'll be a baby waiting for you at the end of it.'

'But you start out so full of hope, don't you, with any fertility treatment? And you try so hard to hold onto that hope – until staying hopeful starts to feel like stupidity rather than optimism. Until staying hopeful starts to feel as though you haven't got a grip on reality any more.'

'Whatever we decide to do next, I think we need to make sure that we go into it with our eyes open. We need to make sure that the *second* that we feel that things aren't working out for us or that we need a break – we knock it on the head or postpone it or whatever. We need to make sure that we don't just carry on regardless, ignoring the effect that it's having on us, ignoring the effect that it's having on our relationship. I don't want to end up ravaged by baby hunger.'

And then I remembered a fertility tracking system that one of my friends had told me about, months before. And I dug out the information that my friend had sent over to me. I dusted off the explanatory accompanying video and Paul and I settled down to watch it. And the video certainly made for some interesting viewing.

The system was based on keeping track of everything that happened during each menstrual cycle – the length and flow of each period, observations about cervical mucus, the timing of intercourse, that kind of thing. And then the observations were charted, on a daily basis, and analysed, on a monthly basis, to detect patterns – like the occurrence of fertile days and the regularity of cycle lengths – and to detect problems like irregular periods and the failure to ovulate. The underlying principle of the fertility tracking system was that if you knew what a normal chart should look like, then you could recognize and solve any problems in an abnormal chart. But the real beauty of the fertility tracking system seemed to be that if an abnormality was detected – and treatment was never offered unless a specific problem had been identified – then the timing of any further tests or of any treatment could be incredibly accurate because there was such a detailed understanding of what was happening on any particular day within each cycle.

Paul and I both decided that it was worthwhile giving it a go and so we set about finding ourselves a practitioner of the approach.

Seconds out, Round Two

As it turned out, finding a practitioner of the fertility tracking approach couldn't have been easier. And our first appointment with him really couldn't have come soon enough. Just a couple of days before our appointment, Paul and I had had the kind of row that we had never had before – a door slamming, plate throwing, angry words spoken kind of row – a row that had blown up over absolutely nothing. Eventually, the fight had left both of us. And, very slowly, we became prepared to leave our respective corners. And then we started to talk.

'I'm dreading our appointment this week,' I said, 'I'm absolutely dreading it. Just the idea of kicking off yet another round of fertility treatment is enough to bring me out in a cold sweat.'

'I'm not exactly keen on the prospect either, you know …'

'It just seems so unfair that we have to go through all of this … this *hassle.* When having babies just seems so easy for other people.'

'I know. If I never heard another pregnancy announcement again – *as long as I lived* – it would be too soon. I'm sick of hearing other people's "happy news". Knowing that they haven't had to endure any of the tests or any of the treatments that we've had to endure.' Paul continued, 'And then, just saying that, makes me feel like an absolute bastard. Knowing that I'm jealous of my friends, that I'm jealous of their happiness ... It's a nightmare, isn't it? You're supposed to be open and honest, these days. You're supposed to be upfront about your feelings. But sometimes, you can't be. Sometimes it's impossible. Because if you told people what you were really thinking, what you were really *feeling*, half of your mates would never speak to you again.'

Until the day of that row – and, actually, during our whole experience of unexplained infertility – I think that Paul and I had been on something of an emotional seesaw together. When one of us had been down, the other one of us had been up. And I had found it frustrating at times. When I had really wanted to do nothing more than wallow in self-pity, Paul had been there, cheering me up and chivvying me along into a better frame of mind. And I am pretty sure that it had been exactly the same for him, too. But on that particular day – when the combination of both of our dark moods had caused the whole emotional seesaw to come crashing down, with us on top of it – it had seemed as though we had had no alternative but to express our deepest emotions, our most unpleasant emotions, our best hidden emotions. We talked about our anger and our disappointment. We talked about our frustration and our hopelessness. We talked about our sadness and our helplessness. And then we talked about how much we loved each other. And then both of us started to feel better. And so we decided to pick ourselves up and dust ourselves off and get ourselves ready for the next round in our quest for a baby.

Cervical Mucus Monitoring for Beginners

I certainly wasn't the oldest woman attempting to conceive using the fertility tracking approach. It turned out that the average age of women using the approach was thirty-six and so I was positively a whippersnapper by comparison. And there were couples using the approach that had been trying for a baby for much longer than Paul and myself. One couple had been trying for a baby for seventeen years. *Seventeen years.* And, harsh as it sounds, I remember hoping that I would have either had a baby or come to terms with *not* having had a baby before I let seventeen years of my life slip on by.

After our first appointment with the fertility tracking practitioner, I did feel as though I was beginning to see some light at the end of the tunnel. The practitioner explained to us that the fertility tracking approach didn't continue indefinitely, that it was basically an eighteen-month course of tracking and treatment and that if a pregnancy could occur, then it would occur within that time frame. And, if a pregnancy didn't occur, then it was back to Plan B. Whatever Plan B turned out to be for Paul and me. Maybe Plan B *was* a couple of attempts at IVF, maybe it was fostering or adoption, maybe it was even attempting to come to terms with a future without kids. But, anyway, it looked as though Paul and I had eighteen months before we even had to think about Plan B.

The practitioner asked both of us a lot of questions. He asked how long we had been trying for a baby. He asked about what tests and what treatments we had had, so far. He asked about my miscarriage. And he asked about my periods. And, when he heard what we had to say, he seemed fairly convinced that the problems that we had been experiencing were caused by a hormonal imbalance. He seemed fairly convinced that the problems were caused by a hormonal imbalance in me – a progesterone deficiency. And he seemed fairly positive that a combination of tracking – to make doubly sure that a progesterone deficiency was, indeed, what the problem was – and treatment – a series of hormone injections – would do the trick for us. And so Paul and I had some hope again.

We left the practitioner's office with a bundle of charts and instructions and colour coded stickers so that I could begin my tracking that very same day. There were little red stickers for period days. There were little green stickers for non-fertile days. And there were little white stickers with babies on them for fertile days. And it was weird, really, because the thing that I found hardest that first month – not being able to have sex until I had got the hang of the fertility tracking system – was also, in many ways, the thing that I found the most liberating. I wanted a baby so badly that the idea of missing an entire month's worth of opportunities to conceive one seemed pretty difficult to get my head around. But there was also this feeling that, for the first time in almost four years, I could just get on with my life instead of thinking, 'Maybe this month is the month ...' I heard two pregnancy announcements that month and I felt nothing but happiness for the bearers of the news. It really did feel as though I had turned a corner.

The Fertility Police

One important element of the fertility tracking approach was some fairly rigorous training on accurate charting methods. I guess that it made sense, really, when it was the charts that formed the basis of any future tests and of any future treatments. And so, in addition to the guidelines that the practitioner had already given us about charting – both face to face and contained in all of the bumph that we had left his office with – Paul and I were required to attend at least one session with a fertility tracking trainer. After we had been tracking for a couple of weeks, just to make sure that we were following all of the instructions, just to make sure that we were doing things right.

I remember feeling pretty upbeat as I got out of bed on the morning of our meeting with the fertility tracking trainer. I felt happy and positive and as though I had not only a good grasp of the charting techniques but also a better understanding of my cycle and my body. We arrived at the trainer's house. And, despite her obvious pregnancy and the fact that if the jumble of toys piled up in her conservatory were anything to go by – she already had at least a couple more children – my buoyant mood continued unabated.

I handed over my chart, fairly sure that I had been following the instructions to the letter. The trainer studied my chart.

The minutes ticked past. And Paul and I waited in silence. I started to get the distinct impression that my chart was going to be handed back to me, with 'could do better' scrawled across it in red pen. And I wasn't far wrong.

'Along the side here, in the date column, we've got 14/3 instead of 14th March.'

I didn't know what to say. I was dumbstruck. I actually thought that she might have been joking, at first, although she looked serious enough.

'We might end up getting confused, you see, about what date we mean.'

The only thing that I was in any danger of getting confused about was the trainer's annoyingly persistent use of the royal 'we'. I tried to stop myself from thinking, 'There are three of us in this relationship ...' Then I felt annoyed. I remember thinking to myself, 'I may be infertile but I'm not a bloody imbecile. I could write the date in French if I wanted to, I could write the date in *Russian*, and I'd still know what date I meant.'

And then she asked me about my wiping habits, when I went to the toilet. And Paul tried – manfully but unsuccessfully – to keep his face straight.

'Now when we go to the loo, do we make sure that we wipe – front to back – twice, on every single visit? To make sure that we get good observations? For our chart?'

'Pretty much, yeah.' I heard myself transforming into a surly teenager.

'Now, Isla, our goal is to do it one hundred per cent of the time, isn't it?'

The trainer didn't seem to be put off by my open hostility or by Paul's barely contained mirth.

'And when we get up for a wee in the night, do we make sure that we pop the light on and wipe – front to back – twice?'

'I don't go to the toilet in the night.'

'But if we *did* go to the toilet in the night, would we make sure that we popped the light on and wiped – front to back – twice?'

Somehow, I managed to resist the powerful urge to shout, 'Exactly which part of "*We* do not go to the toilet in the night" is it that *we* don't understand?' I held my tongue until the lesson was over and Paul and I were, eventually, excused. As soon as we got home, the moment that we had stepped through the front door, I pounced on Paul. And I made love to him. Defiantly. And during our first cycle, during a cycle that was supposed to be nookie free. Ha!

Making a Day of it

Another important element of the fertility tracking approach was carefully timed blood tests. Both Paul and I had breathed a sigh of relief when we realized that the nurse at our local doctor's surgery could carry out the blood tests. Neither of us had wanted to traipse up to the fertility tracking practitioner's office for the injections and we were certainly in no particular hurry to be making a return visit to the trainer's house. The nurse at our local doctor's surgery was a really lovely woman, warm and interested and incredibly supportive. And it was probably just as well. Paul and I were going to be spending a lot of time down at that doctor's surgery. The same blood test had to be carried out on a specific day during the second half of each and every cycle. And only then would we get a clear picture of what was happening with my hormone levels. Only then would we know if my balance of oestrogen and progesterone was as it ought to be.

Paul and I both tried to resign ourselves to the fact that tracking and charting and these monthly blood tests – and the subsequent week-long wait for their results – were, for the foreseeable future, going to become a fairly constant part of our life. And I remembered a really interesting conversation that I had with a woman who seemed incredibly clued up, at a meditation workshop. We had been talking about times of uncertainty in our lives and about waiting for things to happen. And she had told me that, years before, she had made the decision to change her attitude toward waiting. She had changed it from one of frustration and impatience to one of excitement and of curiosity. And she told me that her entire life had improved as a result.

So I decided to apply the wisdom of that woman's thinking to the situation that was facing us. I applied the wisdom of her thinking to our situation of seemingly perpetual waiting – for appointment dates and for test results and for a baby. So Paul and I turned my blood test days into holiday days – albeit holidays with a vaguely unpleasant and uncomfortable five minutes in the middle of them. We would kick off our day by heading to our favourite café for a leisurely brunch, for French toast and lattes and a relaxed hour with the papers before the appointment for my blood test. And then, after my blood test, we would head off for a drive, to somewhere picturesque. When the weather was good, we would drive to the coast or to the lakes or to the mountains. If it was raining, we would visit a local gallery or a bookshop. And we made sure that we turned our waiting into living.

Do Try This at Home

We had been told that, with the fertility tracking approach, it was extremely unlikely to come away with the incredibly frustrating diagnosis of unexplained infertility. And our situation turned out to be no exception. The practitioner's initial stab at a diagnosis, in our very first meeting with him, had been proved right by my blood test results. Although my hormone levels were, as defined by our GP, within the normal range, according to the fertility tracking approach, I had a slight hormonal imbalance. Not quite enough progesterone to get pregnant and, more significantly, not quite enough progesterone to stay pregnant.

I did feel a certain sense of relief that, after four years of trying and failing to have a baby, Paul and I finally had some kind of explanation. I was relieved that a diagnosis of a progesterone deficiency was by no means uncommon. And I was relieved that a progesterone deficiency was treatable, by a series of three injections toward the end of each cycle that could, relatively straightforwardly, be done at home. But I still remember hoping and praying, I still remember crossing my fingers and my toes – a few days after our second meeting with the fertility tracking practitioner – for my period *not* to start. I was hoping that I wouldn't have to have yet more fertility treatment. I was praying that we wouldn't have to do the injections at home. But my hoping and my praying didn't work. And Paul added another string to his bow – the administration of intra-muscular injections.

I hadn't realized just how squeamish I was before, about needles. I could hardly even bring myself to touch them. Paul and I had been told that the more relaxed you managed to be about the injections, the less painful they were. But I could feel myself becoming tense as soon I even thought about the needles, let alone saw them, let alone handled them. And so it seemed to make sense for Paul to play nurse. Years before, one of Paul's older brothers had told him a ghoulish story, about the injection of air being the perfect way to polish someone off. And so, at first, Paul had been paranoid about getting air into my blood stream. At first, he had been paranoid about killing me. He was paranoid about hurting me, too. But, after the first injection, it got much easier for both of us and it got much less painful for me. Paul started to feel more confident and managed to do the injections much more quickly, meaning that I had less time to worry about whether or not the instructions had been followed correctly.

And, that first month, the injections worked. When my blood test results came back, my progesterone levels and my oestrogen levels were textbook perfect, according to the fertility tracking practitioner. So all that remained for me to do was get pregnant.

Late, but Not in a Good Way

We were late for our next scheduled meeting with the fertility tracking practitioner – stuck in traffic – and, consequently, we spent what was left of our allotted hour-long appointment feeling rushed. Feeling as though, yet again, there were more questions than answers. And it wasn't just the questions that had posed themselves in the three months since our last appointment. The most burning of those questions being how many women had managed to conceive using the injections and was I going to be one of those women and, if I was going to be one of those women, then when, when, when?

I felt as though we had been thrown a few curve balls during our appointment, too. There was a throwaway remark about Paul's sperm count being 'not ideal'. And this throwaway remark – one that cast a shadow of uncertainty over everything else that we were doing – was based on the same self semen analysis report that our GP in England had proclaimed as 'normal' just a year or so before. Incredibly, looking back, we didn't even get the chance to ask why. In what way was Paul's sperm count 'not ideal'?

Maybe I was too busy being subjected to a trans-vaginal scan to ask the question, a scan that was required to make sure that the hormone injections I was having weren't causing any cysts on my ovaries. An unbelievably scary-sounding side effect about which, until that point, Paul and I had both been completely and blissfully unaware. And as if the possibility of having ovarian cysts wasn't enough to worry about – for the record, I didn't have them – the scan revealed that I did have a retro inverted uterus. Whatever that meant. And so I spent an anxious couple of hours worrying about the implications of retro inverted uteri until I managed to get to my computer. Until I found out that about 15 per cent of women have one. Until I found out that all that it means is that the uterus is tilted backwards instead of forwards. And that it doesn't usually cause any problems.

Then, toward the end of our appointment, we were told that, despite my first cycle of injections being a success from a hormone-regulating point of view, it would take at least three more cycles before we knew whether this particular course of treatment was the right one for me, the right one for us. And that, in three cycles' time, we may well need to evaluate the situation all over again. I may need even more tests and even more treatment. Different treatment, maybe – the fertility drug, Clomid, was mentioned. And I started to feel frantic again. I started to feel desperate. I didn't *want* to have to wait for another three months. I didn't *want* to have to evaluate the situation all over again. I couldn't bear it. Time was moving on. Another three cycles was another three months closer to the menopause. Another three months closer to a time when my baby making opportunities would be over for good.

I tried incredibly hard to regain my sense of perspective. To remind myself that we all shared a common goal – the fertility tracking practitioner and Paul and me. We all wanted the outcome of the tests and the treatment to be a happy one. We all wanted the outcome of the tests and the treatment to be a pregnancy and, ultimately, a baby. And I tried to tell myself that I was lucky, in lots of ways. That a problem had been identified and that it was being treated and that other women in my situation had been successful in their attempts to achieve a pregnancy. I tried to shake off my growing sense of impatience. I tried to think positively.

Curve Ball

And then I decided – for what seems, now, like the most spurious of reasons – to throw in a curve ball of my own. I had read an article in a women's magazine, an article that was full of tips about what you should do if you were struggling to conceive, about what you should do if you had been trying for a baby for a while, without success. The article said that it could be worthwhile getting yourself – and your partner – checked out for sexually transmitted infections (STIs). And the article had gone on to list a bewildering number of sexually transmitted infections – from gonorrhoea to syphilis to chlamydia – a frightening number of which were without symptoms, and which could cause fertility-related complications, especially for women. The article had described complications like pelvic inflammatory disease – or PID – that could cause high temperatures and chronic pain in the abdomen and in the back, as well as inflammation of the fallopian tubes. And the article had said that that inflammation of the fallopian tubes could lead to permanent scarring, to an increased risk of premature birth, and an increased risk of ectopic pregnancy. And that was if the inflammation hadn't already caused so much damage as to render conception an impossibility. Scary stuff.

By the time I read that magazine article, Paul and I had been together – monogamously – for what was getting close to ten years. And so I was *reasonably* sure that it would just be a formality, getting checked out for sexually transmitted infections, that it would just be another box ticked. But, of course, there was the tiniest element of doubt in my mind. What would happen if I managed to persuade Paul that the tests were worthwhile? What would happen if we decided to get ourselves checked out and the tests found something? What would happen if the tests found something serious? What would happen if the tests found something that wasn't just fertility threatening but life threatening, too? What would happen if the tests found something like HIV-infection? I suppose I knew that, in the long run, it would be better to know about something as serious as HIV/AIDS, that it would be better to face up to those kind of facts. But there was still a certain appeal to keeping one's head firmly buried in the sand – that old adage of 'what you don't know can't hurt you'. Only, of course, with something like HIV-infection, I knew that it *would* be hurting you – secretly and silently and surely – whether you knew about it or not.

Making the decision to make an appointment with our local GUM clinic felt like a pretty monumental one for me. I mulled it over for days before I even mentioned it to Paul. I read and reread the magazine article that had sparked off the whole thing. And I called the GUM clinic's advice line for advice. They seemed to think that I didn't have anything to worry about. There was even the slightest suggestion that I would be wasting both my time and theirs. But they did say that I could make an appointment anyway, if I really thought that it would help me to put my mind at rest. And so I chose my moment, very carefully, and I spoke to Paul. As I had expected, Paul was quite sceptical at first. He was fairly sure that if there had been any problems with either of us, they would have been picked up in the battery of tests to which we had already been subjected. But I explained how I felt about the tests. I explained that because I had read about the problems that STIs could cause for couples, for my own peace of mind, I needed to be sure that it wasn't STIs that were causing problems for us. I just needed to be sure. And so Paul humoured me. He said that he would come with me, down to the GUM clinic, so that we could get ourselves checked out.

The Longest Week of My Life

The week that Paul and I spent waiting for the results of our STI tests seemed to last forever. There were a few blissful moments when I managed to distract myself, when I was able to put all thoughts of our follow-up appointment firmly to the back of my mind, when I didn't feel as though there was something hanging over me – hanging over us – ominously and threateningly. And then the black cloud of doubt would return again, to obliterate the light. What if, what if …

In the end, we made the decision to go for the whole shebang and we had ourselves checked out for every imaginable sexually transmitted infection – from HIV to syphilis. We had blood taken. We had swabs taken. And I am still not sure that Paul will ever quite forgive me for the excruciating pain of a swab down his penis to check for gonorrhoea. And now that all the testing was over, all that we could do was wait – as patiently and as calmly and as optimistically as we could – for our results.

Eventually, after what had felt like the longest week of my life so far, the day of our results appointment dawned. Paul and I drove down to the GUM clinic. We handed over our identification number – no names were exchanged, to protect patient confidentiality. We took our places in the waiting room and we waited. I glanced around, looking for distraction, anything to take my mind off the cliché of nervousness that seemed to have taken hold of my body – the butterflies in my stomach, the vice around my temples, the pounding hammer in my heart. The few magazines that were scattered around the place had seen better days and – irrationally but, I think, explicably – I felt a certain amount of reluctance about handling them. In this waiting room of all waiting rooms. And so I settled back into my chair and I indulged in a spot of people watching.

There were a couple of teenagers. They were sitting directly opposite us and attempting to hide their nervousness behind a flimsy veneer of bravado. They kept nudging each other and sniggering and talking, loudly, about fights that they had been in and about how drunk they had been and about who was sleeping with who. I remember a smartly dressed middle-aged man, sitting beside us, gazing, unblinkingly, down at his immaculately polished shoes. I noticed a wedding ring. Paul kicked me and frowned. I guess I must have been staring.

More people arrived. Some of them had their numbers called almost immediately. They were told their fates behind firmly closed doors and then they left, to face the world.

And then it was our turn.

And, finally, we could breathe again.

Paul and I had been given the all-clear.

Hopes and Hormones

I think I knew, deep down, that the results of our STI tests would come back OK, but I still felt as though I had been given a clean slate, a fresh page. And I felt as though I could turn my attention, whole-heartedly and without distraction, to sorting out my hormonal balance. As though I could focus on meeting the oestrogen and progesterone level targets that had been set for me. And so I was completely unprepared, after my third cycle of hormone injections, for everything to start going so horribly pear-shaped.

I do remember having a bit of a panic when, despite heading rapidly toward the middle of my cycle, there was still no indication that ovulation had occurred. Regular ovulation had been the one thing that I felt my body could be relied upon to do on its own and I certainly didn't want a course of hormone injections to upset that particular apple cart. And so I had breathed a sigh of relief when, later in my cycle than I had anticipated, I had noticed the ovulation indicators that had begun to seem like old friends to me – the abdominal twinge of Mittelschmerz and trademark egg-white cervical mucus.

But then I had a confusing couple of days at the end of my cycle, too. On the day that my period was due, I noticed a spot or two of something dark in my underwear but then that was it, nothing else and certainly not a period. And the days passed with an almost unbearable slowness as I tried, largely unsuccessfully, to steer my mind toward something, anything other than the agony that was maybe-baby speculation. I told myself that if I *was* pregnant, then those dark spots probably weren't the best of signs. Not so many months before, exactly the same kind of dark spotting had heralded the start of my miscarriage. And so I tried to tell myself that I *wasn't* pregnant. And then I argued with myself. I argued with myself because I couldn't remember having any PMT-type symptoms. And the fertility tracking practitioner had told me that in the short term, the hormone injections would probably make those kinds of symptoms worse. And the days carried on dragging by. The speculation – am I pregnant, am I *not* pregnant? – was really starting to get to me. It was becoming nigh on impossible for me to even think about anything else. And so I decided to call my fertility tracking practitioner.

'My period is late, a few days late – and I'm thinking of doing a pregnancy test,' I told him.

'Hold on, hold on,' he said. 'You need to wait a couple more days, at least. A pregnancy test at this stage in your cycle could give you a falsely positive result. It might say that you are pregnant, even if you're not, just because the injections have caused a hormonal surge.'

And I remember thanking God that I had asked the question. The thought of doing a pregnancy test and of the pregnancy test being positive and of Paul and me jumping for joy and then of my period starting, a couple of days later, was one that was just far too painful to bear. And then my period *did* start a couple of days later and I *was* disappointed, of course I was.

I was disappointed every month. But I do remember thinking, 'Hey, life goes on.'

And then Paul and I got back the results of my blood tests – the blood tests that monitored my progesterone levels and my oestrogen levels.

Throwing in the Towel

The blood test results revealed that my oestrogen level had soared and that my progesterone level had plummeted. That was exactly the opposite effect to the one that I wanted, exactly the opposite effect to the one that I *needed*. Excessive oestrogen levels meant bad skin and a heightened risk of ovarian cysts and even breast cancer. Insufficient progesterone levels meant more and worse PMT symptoms and a much greater likelihood of miscarriage. And a combination of excessive oestrogen levels and insufficient progesterone levels meant that there was no baby for Paul and me. Again.

It seemed to me that I had a lot of thinking to do – a lot of decisions to make and not just about improving our chances of having a baby. I needed to think about what was best for me, too. I needed to make some decisions about what I thought was best for my own health and well-being, about what I thought was best for my own *sanity*. And I felt scepticism creeping in again. I felt scepticism creeping in about the usefulness of the hormone injections that had been prescribed for us by our fertility tracking practitioner. I remembered that our GP had told us that there was nothing wrong with my hormone levels. I remember thinking that, presumably, they knew *something* about fertility. And anyway, I reminded myself, I may only have been using the hormone injections for three months but it wasn't as though they appeared to be working. It seemed that the injections were turning a minor hormonal imbalance if, indeed, there had been any hormonal imbalance at all, into a major one. And I realized that I was worried about the long-term health implications of that.

'I just don't know what to do for the best. My gut instinct is telling me to put a stop to this treatment. But, in a way, I'm *scared* to put a stop to it.' My fear wasn't surprising, not really. Our fertility tracking practitioner had told us in no uncertain terms that if we didn't manage to get my hormonal 'problem' sorted out, even IVF wouldn't work for us. He had told us that in the unlikely event of my getting pregnant, naturally or otherwise, it would end in miscarriage. Talk about fear selling.

'Do you remember that thing we read?' Paul asked me, 'About hope being one of the most important things that fertility specialists can pass on to their patients?'

'Course I do ... But I've got to the stage where everything about me – my thoughts and my words and the way that I behave – is screaming "Hopeless!" Again.'

'It's time to throw in the towel, isn't it?'

'I think it is. I think this time it's time to throw it in permanently, though.'

'Enough is enough, eh?'

The Men in White Coats

'Do you feel the same way that I do?'

'I don't know, honey, give me a clue.'

'Do you feel as though our life is finally our own again?'

'Yeah, I do. I feel relieved. And I feel light. In fact, I feel exactly the same way that I did when we were in England, when we'd made the decision to knock *that* lot of fertility treatment on the head.'

'Me too. And so why did we bother putting ourselves through all of that again?'

'What do you mean?'

'When we both felt so great, after stopping our fertility treatment in England; when we felt so light and so relieved and all of those other wonderful things. And then when we'd just got a brand new life for ourselves, in Ireland ...' I thought, for a moment, about what exactly it was that I was trying to say, 'Why was it that less than a year after we'd stopped one lot of fertility treatment we were in such a mad rush to sign up for another lot?'

'Well, because we want a baby, I suppose. And because we'd started to feel as though time was running out for us ... And because we felt as though we needed to *do* something.'

'Yes. And so went trotting along to the experts, because *doctor knows best.*'

And I really don't think that Paul and I had been out of the ordinary, in doing that and in thinking that. I think that most people in the West have been programmed to rely – and, scarily, often unquestioningly – on the opinions and the judgements and the *pronouncements* of the medical profession. It is as though we look to the medical professionals for wisdom and insights into our own bodies, as though we look to them to *provide* us with wellness. We look to doctors and to chemists, to specialists and to prescription drugs for solutions to all of our health problems.

'I do still find it weird, you know, looking back.'

'Find what weird?'

'Well, the way that I just sort of rolled over when it started to look as though we weren't going to be able to have kids. The way that I just rolled over and let the so-called *specialists* do whatever they saw fit with me.'

'Yeah, I suppose …'

'Before all this happened, you could count on one hand the amount of times that I'd been to the doctor during my entire adult life. And I've never been a pill popper. Not even with just over-the-counter stuff. If I ever get a headache, I always try to work out *why*. Am I tired or am I stressed? Have I been doing too much? Have I been working too hard? Have I been drinking too much coffee? Am I just plain hung over? I've always tried to establish the *cause* of any particular ailment so that I can do something about that rather than …'

' … just treating the symptoms,' Paul chipped in. That particularly self-righteous monologue must have been a firm favourite in my repertoire.

'OK, smart arse … I suppose that not being able to have a baby rocked the foundations of what I *thought* I knew about my own body. Not being able to have a baby made me feel helpless. It made me feel *hopeless*.'

And I think that because of that overwhelming sense of helplessness, because of that overwhelming sense of *hopelessness*, I had had no choice but to look elsewhere for help and for hope. And because I really needed to believe that someone somewhere had the answer, that someone somewhere had the solution to our fertility problems, I had chosen to look to the medical professionals – to the doctors and to the specialists. And I had started to see them as all knowing, as all powerful, as *omnipotent*. So I had lurched from treatment to treatment – from fertility drugs to Intra Uterine Insemination to hormone injections – in my increasingly desperate quest to conceive. And I had done it all blindly. I had done it all almost unthinkingly. I had done it all because somebody in a white coat had told me that it was the right thing to do.

As I looked back over the four years that Paul and I had been trying for our baby, all of the faces of the people in the white coats – the doctors and the specialists, the gynaecologists and the consultants – seemed to blur, dizzyingly and confusingly, into one. I remembered fragments of conversations from what, looking back, seemed like an almost endless series of appointments.

Over the past four years I'd been told that there was no physical reason why Paul and I hadn't been able to have a baby. And then I'd been told that there *was* a reason, that there *must* be a reason, that it was simply a case of tracking down the reason.

I'd been told that my hormone levels were fine, they were normal and there was nothing at all for me to worry about. And then I was told that my hormone levels were *abnormal*, that they were inadequate, that I was deficient in some crucial-for-conception way.

I'd been told that, at the end of the day, there was always IVF. And then I was told that IVF wasn't going to be an option for me, that in the unlikely event that IVF *did* work for me, it would end in miscarriage.

I was told that I needed to relax, to forget about having a baby for a while, to put it to the back of my mind. And I'd been told that I needed to focus; that I needed to pop a pill, have a blood test, inject hormones, not to mention told to 'have intercourse' on different and quite specific days throughout my cycle.

And the more I looked back, the more I found I couldn't quite remember who had said what or when. The more I looked back, the more it seemed that the only thing that the people in the white coats had in common with each other was their indifference.

'Do you remember that article? The one about the woman who was in charge of fertility policy for the NHS?'

'The one who said that there's more to life than having children? The one who said that there are worse things in life than *not* having children?'

'Yeah. When it was really easy for her to say that. Because she'd already *got* kids ... But just lately, though, I've started to think that maybe she was right, in a way. Maybe there *are* worse things in life than not having kids. It's just that when you're trying to make your way through the whole traumatic experience of infertility, of failed fertility treatment, of mis-carriages – it really doesn't feel that way.'

'I know what you mean. A lot of the time, over the last few years, I've felt as though not having kids was the very worst thing that life could have thrown at us ...'

'I know. And sometimes I think that it would have made the world of difference for both of us – just once – to have been treated by somebody who at least *tried* to understand that.'

You're Not Alone

There had been times when it had seemed really important for both Paul and myself to feel as though we weren't alone, as though we weren't the only couple in the entire world who were trying to live through the heartache of involuntary childlessness. Friends of ours had done their best to understand what we were going through. But, if I am being honest, I really don't think that it is *possible* to truly and totally empathize with another person unless you have, at some stage in your own life, found yourself in exactly the same situation. And even those friends of ours who *had* been in exactly the same situation, even those friends of ours who had had to undergo fertility treatment themselves, seemed to forget – almost as soon as they had been successful in their efforts and certainly as soon as they had had their babies – just how desperate and hopeless and worthless and sad that the experience of infertility had made them feel. So Paul and I had found a support group for ourselves, a support group for couples who still were in the same situation as us.

The support group organized regional meetings and social activities; they provided a regular newsletter and access to a confidential advice line; they lobbied for investment into medical research and they gave couples experiencing fertility problems a voice. But, more important than any of those things, the sheer number of members that the support group attracted helped Paul and me to realize that we weren't alone, that there were other people out there who knew exactly how we felt. We didn't attend any of the group's meetings and neither one of us was particularly keen on the idea of the social activities.

'Doesn't going ten pin bowling with a complete stranger – just because they can't have kids either – strike you as just a little bit weird?'

'Totally. It's like, *"Look what fun us crazy kid-less kids are having!"'*

But I looked forward to receiving my copies of the newsletter and, as soon as I did receive them, I would read them from cover to cover. There was always something in them that struck a chord with me, there was always something in them that made me think, 'God, yes. I know *exactly* how you feel.'

One woman had written a short article for the newsletter, to share her feelings about Christmas gift giving. She had described how, for years, she had exchanged Christmas gifts with her friends. And she had described how those Christmas gifts had always been just a small token, just a gesture. But then her friends had started to have children, one after the other. And, as the years had passed, the woman had found herself buying more and more presents – for her friends and for their partners, for babies number one and two, for babies number three and four – while she had continued to receive the one, small token from each of her friends. And the woman had described how that had made her feel. Short-changed and hard done by, initially, and then, later, childish and petty.

And, at first, I thought that childish and petty was damn right. I thought that her reaction was almost Scrooge-like. Bah, humbug. But then I remembered how I had felt, on one particular birthday of mine.

'Do you think that I'm being petty?'

'It's your birthday you can be whatever you want to be.'

'I feel *disgruntled*. Two of my friends have put birth announcements and photographs of their newborns in with my birthday card – in the *same* envelope. They haven't even forked out for a different envelope let alone another stamp. And they couldn't even wait a day or two more so that I didn't feel as though I was having my nose rubbed in my own infertility and on my birthday, of all days.'

And so it was reassuring, reading other women's stories in the support group's newsletters. It was reassuring to know that I wasn't the only woman in the world who was thinking deep and dark and *petty* thoughts.

Moving the Goal Posts

I looked back over the years that Paul and I had been trying for our baby and I lost count of the number of newspaper articles that I had read in my seemingly endless quest to find a solution to our fertility problems. I had read magazine articles, I had pored over books in the library and I had searched the Internet. Tirelessly looking for answers, tirelessly looking for solutions. And, despite my very best efforts, I don't think that I had ever really found any. I had managed to gather information about the mind-boggling array of fertility treatments that were available. I had managed to identify – and fret about – a million and one fertility-impacting ailments. But I had never managed to find the one thing that I was *really* looking for. I don't think that I even knew what it was, not until very much later. Because what I was looking for was incredibly difficult to find. I was looking for peace of mind. For a peaceful and accepting and *gentle* state of mind. One where I could truthfully say that life would be great if Paul and I had a baby together but that it would be great if we didn't have a baby together too.

And then I started to think about the bewildering variety of alternative therapies and remedies that I had tried. I thought about how, instead of just relaxing and enjoying what those very different experiences could offer me, I had turned my sessions of yoga and meditation, of reflexology and homeopathy into something goal focused; into something that was focused, and almost exclusively, on our goal of having a baby. And any other benefits that I might have experienced from the treatments were pushed into the background; any other benefits were quickly dismissed as unimportant, as insignificant. If I had failed yet again to reach my goal of getting pregnant, then as far as I was concerned, the treatment had failed too.

But the funny thing was that, despite all of that, I did actually buy into the philosophies that underpinned so many of the mind and body and spirit therapies. I could see there was logic behind them. I could see that it made sense to provide the body with whatever support it needed, be that relaxation or improved nutrition or positive thinking or whatever, in order to heal itself. And I could see that it made sense to aim to heal the entire body and not just the part where any particular symptom had been experienced. I could understand the powerful influence of the mind – on both a conscious level and an unconscious level – on the physical symptoms that are experienced within the body. And I could recognize that the type of symptoms that I was experiencing, symptoms like a continued inability to conceive, could be caused within the body as a whole. Perhaps by blocked or unbalanced energy flows. That they could be caused by less than positive emotional states and by negative thinking, by unexpressed emotions and by unresolved issues. But I had found that, for me, there had been a price to pay for believing in all of those things.

'I just think that things would have been so much easier for us if we knew that our infertility was caused by something straightforward. If it was caused by something cut and dried, by something mechanical and medical.' I elaborated, 'If it was caused by something like faulty fallopian tubes, for example.'

'How so?'

'Well not knowing what's caused our infertility has made me question *everything*. The not knowing has made me look at almost every aspect of our life and ask, is it that? Is it *that* that's stopping us from having a baby? I've questioned our lifestyle and our diet, our stress levels and our exposure to toxins, our alcohol intake and our attitudes ... You name it, basically and I've speculated about it.'

'Well we definitely live a healthier and happier life than we did four years ago so maybe all that speculation hasn't necessarily been a bad thing ...'

'Maybe not ... But what *is* definitely a bad thing is the way that over the last four years, I've blamed myself and *tortured* myself. I've asked myself why, why, why. Why haven't I been able to have a baby? What have I been doing wrong? What have I done to deserve infertility? If there really is such a thing as a mind and body connection, then why have *my* mind and body refused, so stubbornly and persistently, to cooperate with each other?'

So, counterproductive to the underlying principles of alternative therapies – and not to mention counterproductive to the good old fashioned practice of cutting yourself some slack – I would give myself a hard time if I let myself get tired or stressed, if I let myself get angry or upset, if I didn't think positively one hundred per cent of the time. I would beat myself up for not being perfect. I would beat myself up for not being *pregnant*.

After Paul and I had given up on the fertility tracking approach, I made the decision to take some time out for myself, some time out with no ulterior motive, to take some time out with no underlying baby agenda. I had realized, and not before time, that it really was time to take care of myself and to treat myself well and to listen – and respond – to *all* of the messages that I was receiving from my mind and my body and my spirit. And not just the messages that were about conception, pregnancy and babies. It was time for me to take the first few steps on a very different sort of journey, the first few steps on a journey to find the peaceful and accepting and gentle state of mind for which I had been searching for years, if not my entire adult life.

A Few Small Steps and, at the Same Time, a Giant Leap

I invested in a small library of books to help me on the first few steps of my journey. I chose books that I thought would provide me with the resources and the support that I needed in order to find my own wisdom. Books that I thought would help me to regain my sense of balance, of equilibrium. Books that would help me to shake off the overwhelming feelings of failure and hopelessness, of sadness and desperation that had gradually started to envelop me over the years that Paul and I had been trying for our baby. And I made the decision that whatever I chose to do in the future, I would do it first and foremost because it felt good for me, because it felt like the right thing to do and not just because I thought that there was an outside chance of a baby at the end of it.

I decided to work toward changing the way that I did things, too. I decided to work toward changing the way that I prioritized things. In the past, I would always feel this compulsion to get my chores out of the way before I could let myself concentrate on anything speculative, on anything fun and certainly before I could let myself concentrate on anything life changing. And then I would make excuses for myself. I would attempt to justify my behaviour. I would tell myself that the house *had* to be clean and tidy before I started working on anything else. And I would tell myself that it was because I preferred to work on the really important stuff in a clear and uncluttered environment and with a clear and uncluttered mind. But, deep down, I knew that the reality was different. And time after time it seemed that the chores would expand, that they would *multiply,* to fill the time available. And, time after time, the life changing stuff would remain untouched.

And so, as I took the first few steps on my journey, I started to feel as though I was on the brink of something really quite wonderful, something that I couldn't quite define, something that I couldn't quite *describe,* but something that was really quite wonderful nonetheless.

The First Step on the Road toward Understanding Myself

The weeks passed and I started to dip, just tentatively at first, into a selection of the books from my new and rapidly growing library. It felt incredibly liberating to be setting out on a journey that was more about self-awareness and acceptance than about clearly defined goals. And it felt exhilarating to be setting out on a journey that had no clearly defined end point; to be setting out on a journey where I got the feeling that each and every step I took would be a destination in itself.

Most of the books that I had chosen to pore over were in agreement about the fundamental principles of the alternative therapies that I had already experienced, alternative therapies like hypnotherapy and homeopathy. The books described how all of our emotions whether we are conscious of them or not and whether we express them or not can have a physical effect on the body. The books explained that just because you *say* that you're not angry, for example, it doesn't necessarily mean that you really *aren't* angry. And the books explained that the energy that was generated from unexpressed emotions has to go somewhere; that the energy from unexpressed emotions, from *suppressed* emotions, can be stored in the body with potentially damaging consequences. And I started to think about all of the emotions that I had been suppressing over the years, particularly in the four years that Paul and I had been trying for our baby.

I remembered how I would swallow down the anger that I felt when other people, especially my friends and my family, made hurtful or tactless remarks to me. I would say, 'It's OK, I know what you mean.' When, quite often, it wasn't and I didn't.

And I would be reluctant to acknowledge my totally human and completely understandable feelings of bitterness and of jealousy as they almost inevitably arose when friend after friend and relative after relative called to tell me that they were pregnant. I wasn't comfortable about acknowledging those emotions because they made me feel guilty, because they made me feel ashamed. And my friends and my family were all lovely people; they would have done their best to understand if only I had been brave enough to be honest with them.

I could have said to them, 'Look, I am absolutely delighted for you but, at the same time, I'm really sad for me. I feel frustrated and impatient and inadequate because I still haven't had a baby, because I'm *still* not pregnant. And I'm a little bit scared that, when your baby comes along, you won't want to – or be able to – spend quite so much time with me. I'm scared that, gradually, we'll drift apart because we just don't have enough in common any more.' But of course I never did, I was never quite that honest. And instead, upon hearing pregnancy announcement after pregnancy announcement, I would squeal down the phone, 'Oh my God! What exciting news!' And I would wonder why my throat ached and my stomach hurt and my head throbbed as I put down the phone.

But the thought of being consistently open and honest about my feelings and not just when I had hit rock bottom, like the time Paul and I lost our baby, had always made me feel incredibly vulnerable before. It was as though I was scared of the depth of my own emotions. I wondered what would happen if I let myself acknowledge my feelings of bitterness and disappointment, of frustration and helplessness, of loneliness and inadequacy, of jealousy and sadness. I wondered what would happen if, once I had opened those emotional floodgates, I couldn't close them again. But on my new journey and with my books to support me and to point me in the right direction, I was feeling brave. What was the worst thing that could happen to me?

Letting Myself Cry

Guided by a series of exercises in one of my books – and aware that recognition of any particular issue was half way along the road to resolving it – I decided that I was going to acknowledge my sadness. I decided that I was going to let myself cry. And my tears were surprisingly ready; they were surprisingly close to the surface. I cried tears of bitterness and sadness. I cried tears of loneliness and hopelessness. I cried tears of anger and frustration. I cried because the thought of never having a child of my own still filled me with such a deep and immense sense of sadness. I cried at the unfairness of it all. I cried because the only pregnancy that we had achieved together – Paul and me – had ended in miscarriage. And I cried because, deep down, I still blamed myself for that. I cried because I didn't think that I was ever going to experience for myself one of the most basic and primal and *joyful* of human functions and I cried because just thinking about that made me feel such an overwhelming sense of loss. I cried because not having a baby sometimes felt as though it was a form of punishment because I wasn't good enough, because I wasn't perfect enough. And I cried because the person who was really punishing me was myself.

I cried until I really couldn't cry any more and then – as my tears subsided and eventually dried – I felt cleansed and refreshed. I felt as though I had been liberated from a deep well of sadness that had been threatening to drown me. I had provided myself with just the type of bereavement counselling that I had been silently crying out for, for so very many years. And I realized that I had taken the most difficult step of any journey – the first one.

Denial, Blame and Trying to Be Perfect

I continued to work through a series of exercises from my books and my journey began to take me to deeply buried parts of myself. I started to uncover feelings and beliefs about which, before, I had been only barely aware. I realized that illness, for example, made me acknowledge the vulnerability of human beings, that it made me acknowledge the fine line between sickness and health, that it made me acknowledge the fragility and the precariousness and the impermanence of life. And I realized that illness scared me. And as I dug a little deeper, I became aware and was – rather surprised – that I would transform that sense of fear into one of anger and of frustration and even into one of intolerance when friends and family and other people around me became ill.

When other people became ill – when *Paul* became ill even – I would very quickly start to feel impatient with them. And on the rare occasions that I would actually allow myself to accept that they *were* ill – that they were not just being hypochondriacs, they were not just making it up – my sympathy would be in fairly limited supply. And, irrationally, I would blame them. I would imagine that, somehow, they had managed to bring their illnesses on to themselves. It was as though I couldn't cope with the reality that sometimes the people closest to me *would* become ill and that, quite often, they would become ill for no apparent reason.

And I recognized that I had an almost boastful approach to my own, usually robust, health. I recognized that this boastfulness would become particularly pronounced when I was at work. I would proudly tell my colleagues, 'Do you know, I can't remember the last time I had a cold' or 'I'm not an upset stomach sort of person.' And, quite often, I *wouldn't* be ill for months and months on end but then, as soon as I was away from work for any length of time, for a summer holiday or for the Christmas break, I would find myself with a streaming cold; when I didn't feel the pressure to be super-human, when I felt as though I could let my guard down, when I could allow myself to be vulnerable. And I suppose that finding it difficult to get pregnant and then losing a baby didn't quite fit with the super-human standards for health and wellness that I had for myself. It made me feel as though I was weak. It made me feel as though I was sub-standard in some way, as though I was faulty. It made me feel ashamed because I was less than perfect.

And perfection did seem to be such a hard taskmaster. Although Paul and I had always known that we wanted to have children together, at some stage, like so many other couples that we knew, we had also wanted everything else in our lives to be as close to perfect as possible before we would even consider *trying* for our baby. We had wanted our children to have a healthy life and a happy life, we had wanted them to have everything that their hearts desired; we had wanted – for them and for us – everything to be *perfect.* And I thought back to the day when Paul and I had made the decision to start trying for our baby. I thought back to the list of questions that we had asked ourselves, all those years before.

Would we be good parents? Would we be 'good enough' parents? Were we ready for the responsibility of a tiny human being relying on us for absolutely everything? Had we grown up enough yet ourselves? How would we feel about putting our social life on hold for a year (or for five years or for ten years or for twenty years)? Would I ever be able to get into a pair of size ten jeans again? Would I ever be able to spend hours in the bath, smothered in beauty treatments, sipping white wine and leafing through glossy magazines? How would our relationship be affected? Would we have any energy left for each other after disturbed nights and feeding on demand? Would Paul still fancy me after watching me give birth? Would I ever even want him to fancy me again? What about our careers? Were we stable enough, financially, to have a baby? Could we cope with such a huge drop in income? Would I be able to or want to pick up where I left off after maternity leave? Would Paul feel overwhelmed by financial responsibility? Pressurized into being the sole breadwinner? Was our house big enough? Was it child friendly enough? Was it in the right catchment area for the best possible local schools?

And I wondered if it was humanly possible ever to be able to answer all of those questions positively and confidently. I wondered if it was even *desirable*. What the future holds is an unknown quantity for all of us, no matter what steps we might take to try and influence it and, surely, that is part of the joy and the mystery of life.

But of course it's easy to say all of that now, looking back. When Paul and I had started trying for our baby, I had felt very differently. I had wanted my experience of motherhood to be idyllic. I had wanted it to be perfect. I had wanted it to be how I imagined motherhood *would* have been in the good old days. A happy and contented mum with a healthy brood of kids; floury hands and warm, sunny kitchens filled with the smell of home baking; hugs and kisses and cakes iced with the word 'Daddy' for the happy worker. And then I had spoken to my own grandmother. I had asked her about how things had been when my mum was a little girl. And I had got a reality check, a wake-up call and my fond but erroneous imaginings about the good old days had disappeared in a puff of smoke.

My grandmother told me that like the vast majority of her contemporaries she had had to carry on working after my mum was born. She told me that she had relied on one of her sisters to look after my mum, and that her sister had taken in children for quite a few of the local working mothers. My grandmother told me that she had had to juggle being a mother and being a wife and being an employee and being *herself* in exactly the same way that my contemporaries were doing in the noughties. And so it seemed that even the good old days were far from perfect, too.

Looking for the Silver Linings

And then one day, I decided to make a list for myself. I decided to make a list of all the positive things my involuntary childlessness had brought me. At first I just sat there, with a blank piece of paper in front of me, unable to think of a single positive thing about our childlessness. And then I remembered a technique I had read about, in one of my books, a technique that could help to turn thinking around, one that could help to turn negative statements into positive ones. And the technique was simple. All that you had to do was decide carefully about the language that you used, to choose positive words instead of negative ones. So rather cornily problems weren't problems any more, they were opportunities. And life was no longer a struggle, it was exciting, it was an adventure, it was full of possibilities. So I decided to try out the technique for myself, to give my own list a kick-start.

At first, the things that I wrote down were really quite muddled and it was difficult to see where the negativity ended and where anything positive began. At first, I wrote things like:

I have always wanted to be a bit different, to stand out from the crowd. Words like ordinariness and routine, anonymity and mainstream are enough to bring me out in a cold sweat. And so maybe not having a baby is what makes me different, maybe not having a baby is what sets me apart from everybody else.

If I never have children of my own, I will never have to face up to the possibility of being a less-than-perfect parent. I will never have to worry about the reality of parenthood. I can choose to focus on the opinions of other people, 'It is such a shame that Paul and Isla can't have kids, they really would be *wonderful* parents.' I will never have to worry about not being able to live up to that hype.

If Paul and I had a baby when we had first started trying, we would still be living in England, stuck in jobs that were less than rewarding in every way other than financially, handing over our children to child-minders so that we could maintain the two incomes required to cover our enormous mortgage and trying – desperately and miserably – to keep up with a ubiquitous Jones family to whom we could barely relate.

And then I surprised myself. Once I had started the *process* of writing, a stream of pure and positive thoughts just seemed to flow out of me and onto the paper in front of me.

I feel infinitely more mature and more grounded and more balanced than I did four years ago, when Paul and I first started trying for our baby. My understanding of myself and my dreams, my hopes and my fears, my strengths and my weaknesses is better than it has ever been before. I have been provided with a unique and valuable opportunity to really get to know myself inside and out.

If Paul and I *are* ever lucky enough to have a child of our own or if we decide to foster a child or to adopt, in the future, I feel as though I have the emotional intelligence to really enjoy the experience of parenting, to have with my children the fulfilling and rewarding and loving relationships that I desire.

And, for the first time in my life, I am living for *now*. Not for a future moment when x or y or z may or may not happen. I am enjoying the moment. Finally, I have learnt how to make the most out of each and every day.

Becoming Human

With a sense of relief, I realized that I was finally able to smile, if not laugh out loud, at some of the ridiculously tactless comments that people had made to Paul and me over the years that we had been trying for our baby. I felt a sense of relief because it hadn't always been that way – far from it. At one particularly painful stage Paul and I had even bought little notebooks, we had called the notebooks our 'Tactless Logs' and we would scribble down howler after howler as a much needed way of letting off some steam.

'You really can't expect other people to put off having their families, you know, just because you and Paul can't have kids.'

'God, it was horrible phoning you to tell you that I was pregnant. If I'm being honest, I put it off and I phoned absolutely everyone else first.'

'*Getting* pregnant has always been more of a worry for me. I only have to think about babies – I only have to *look* at a baby – and I'm pregnant again.'

'I bet that if you and Paul split up and both started trying to have a baby with your *new* partners, the pair of you would end up with babies almost straightaway.'

And I remember a friend who used to use the words 'impotent' and 'infertile' as though they were interchangeable, as though they had the same meaning. And I would cringe every time our conversations headed towards that particular danger zone. I would hope and pray that Paul was out of earshot, that his sense of masculine sexuality at least could remain intact.

I remember a different friend, a heavily pregnant one, showing me drawer after drawer of tiny baby clothes – little socks and little t-shirts and little vests. And I remember doing my absolute best to make all of the right noises. Doing my absolute best to appear happy and to appear interested. But I also remember wondering what would happen in a slightly different, but no less comparable situation to that one? What would happen if the situation involved a rich friend and a poor friend? Would the rich friend really expect the poor friend to – happily and interestedly – coo over their much healthier-looking bank statements? Hardly.

My experience of involuntary childlessness taught me that words can – and do – hurt just as much as the sticks and stones of the playground rhyme. I lost count of the amount of times that I was asked by friends and by family, by colleagues and even by people that I had only just met, 'Don't you want children?' And I remember thinking that unless you were incredibly and pathologically tactless you wouldn't ask somebody who was overweight, 'Don't you want to be slim?'

But I was as guilty as the next person. I had done exactly the same thing myself, long before babies had crept on to the agenda for Paul and me. I remember a woman who I used to work with, when I was in my early twenties, when I was fresh out of university. My colleague must have been in her late thirties – she had certainly been married for a good few years – and, in response to what I realize now was an incredibly tactless and probably extremely hurtful question, she had told me that she didn't ever want to have children. And I was forever asking her why. I was forever bugging her about it. For some reason, I just wouldn't let the subject drop. And then years later, long after I had left that particular company – eager to move on to bigger and better things – I had heard that she was pregnant. After numerous miscarriages and several failed attempts at IVF. And I felt bad, of course I did, I felt guilty. But it wasn't until I experienced infertility for myself that I really *understood*.

And remembering how I had been with that work colleague, all those years before, made me realize that it *is* hard for other people. It is hard for other people to do the right thing and to say the right thing no matter how badly they would like to be able to do just that. It is hard for them because most people haven't had to endure the emotional – and sometimes physical – pain of infertility first hand. It is hard because, unless they have a particularly vivid imagination, it is virtually impossible for other people to appreciate just what exactly you are going through. And so, as the years passed, I gradually learned to see the innocence in other people's words and in other people's behaviour. I knew that my friends and my family and even the acquaintances, the relative *strangers*, who interrogated me about our baby making plans wanted Paul and me to be happy. And I knew that it upset them, – the ones that knew the truth, that Paul and I hadn't been able to have a baby. And so, as the years passed, I learned how to cut them some slack.

'Do you remember when we got that pregnancy announcement by email?'

'When your friend told you that she was pregnant and then asked if there was any baby news from our end?'

'That's the one. And I was furious, remember? My first reaction was to email her back and say, "Oh my God, I'm so sorry. It must have completely slipped my mind. I've successfully given birth to a pair of twins since our last email ...'

'How could I forget?'

'And then I forced myself to take a deep breath and consider the facts. I knew that my friend was telling me her news via email because, that way, she could be more certain of saying the right thing. Because that way she could re-read what she had written rather than blurting something out over the phone and offending me. And I knew that she was asking about our baby news because she, so badly, wanted me to be pregnant too.'

And when I started to look for the innocence in what other people said and did, all of a sudden the world, seemed like a brighter and a happier and an infinitely more loving place.

Relaxation, Japanese Style

I was incredibly proud of all of the work that I had done. I was incredibly proud of just how far I had travelled. So I decided that I was going to treat myself; I was going to celebrate my success. My yoga teacher had recommended a shiatsu massage therapist who practised in our local area and so I put my name down for a course of three massages.

Shiatsu is an ancient Japanese healing therapy and, similar to the alternative therapies that I had already experienced, it is based on the principle that disease occurs as a result of blocked or unbalanced energy. So to regulate the flow of life energy and to stimulate the healing of the body and the mind, the shiatsu therapist uses their hands and their feet, their elbows and their knees in order to manipulate and to massage the body's acupuncture points.

Before we could get to the massage bit of the treatment, my shiatsu therapist had had the usual questions to ask me about my diet and my lifestyle, about my sleeping patterns and my periods, about my stress levels and my general health. And then, rather unusually and certainly unexpectedly, she had asked me if she could take a look at my tongue. Happily, as it turned out, my tongue was pink and clean and healthy-looking and certainly didn't display any of the signs of imbalance for which the therapist was looking. And so we could get down to the serious business of relaxation.

My therapist asked me to lie on my back, at first, on a mattress on the floor. I closed my eyes and breathed deeply while she worked on my body with firm and decisive movements. I rolled over, when asked to do so, as the therapist continued with her work. And then out of nowhere – I burst out laughing. And it was a proper belly laugh – inexplicable and uncontrollable and yet filled with joy and mirth. And my therapist explained that that wasn't uncommon. She said that people experienced many different reactions in their first few sessions of shiatsu, some people laughed, some people cried, some people just felt an incredible sense of calmness and serenity. And as my laughter eventually subsided, I relaxed back into the soft mattress and tried to visualize my life's energy flowing smoothly and freely around my body. I felt healthy and I felt hopeful but, more importantly, I felt *happy*.

Letting Life In

Less than a year ago, I was living in England. I was going through the motions, leading a life that was to all intents and purposes successful. I was a home owner, I had a very nice house, thank you very much. I had a good job, a well paid one, a relatively secure one. And I had a brand new company car. Fear stopped me from letting any of it go, and fear stopped me from opening up my life to anything new.

I was frightened that if made the mistake of selling one house without, immediately, buying another one, that would be it. I would be off the property ladder. I would be committing financial *suicide*. I imagined that house prices would rocket and that I would be no better off than a first-time buyer by the time I had decided to climb back onto the property ladder. I imagined, God forbid, that I might even end up with a smaller house, a less *prestigious* house, than the one that I had sold. And that wasn't the way that property ownership was supposed to work. I was supposed to be constantly striving for something slightly bigger and something slightly better, something slightly more expensive and something with slightly more difficult Joneses to keep up with. Never mind selling up, never mind renting for a year or two, never mind giving yourself a bit of breathing space.

I was frightened that if I made the mistake of resigning from my job and without another one to go to – I may as well kiss goodbye to any future financial security. I imagined that I would struggle to get another, equivalent, job. I imagined that, at interviews, I would be hard pushed to explain away the gap in gainful employment on my CV. And I imagined myself having to take a step down, having to take a step back. I imagined that I would never drive a brand new company car again.

I was frightened that I would lose my identity. I was a well-paid marketing manager. I drove a BMW. I lived in a barn conversion in a prestigious little development with just the right postcode. What would I be if I left it all behind? Unemployed and living in rented accommodation. And, without kids, I couldn't even legitimately call myself a housewife. Not really. So it wasn't exactly fear of the unknown that was holding me back, it was fear of the *known*. I could imagine my fate all too vividly. Penniless and homeless and jobless and childless. But Paul and I made the decision to make the leap anyway.

The Future is Bright and the Here and Now is Pretty Good, Too

And, now, I wonder why it took the two of us so long. I wonder why it took us so long to grab what courage we had with both pairs of hands and make the leap. Why it took us so long to make the decision to leave it all behind – all of the material things that we had managed to accumulate, the financial security, the career paths that we had carved out for ourselves. And sometimes, when I look back, I feel as though fate just seemed to take over, as though it had had enough of our dithering, enough of our indecision. I feel as though our new life just started to *happen*, almost of its own volition. I feel as though one day we were just going through the motions, treading water, passing time. And then the next day – at a time when I had least expected it, at a time when our childlessness had rendered me lethargic, immobile – Paul and I had taken the giant leap that we needed to take in order to actually start *living*.

And we are living a pretty good life, now, Paul and me.

A couple of months ago, we bought ourselves a little whitewashed cottage, five minutes' walk from an absolutely beautiful and usually deserted beach. And most afternoons,

Paul and I head down to that beach together. And as we walk, we talk. And we breathe in the sea air and the changing seasons and the contentment and the joy and the security that we feel in each other's presence.

On other afternoons, we will potter for hours in our garden. We will scratch our heads, trying to work out just what exactly it is that we are supposed to be doing with our three quarters of an acre. The vision that I had had of myself – wafting around a delightful cottage garden in a long and floaty skirt, gathering long stemmed yellow roses, maybe cultivating an organic vegetable or two – has yet to materialize. And we have talked, and really quite seriously, of plumping for the 'rustic, unkempt field' look for our garden. We have talked about getting ourselves a donkey, or a goat, to help us to keep the grass below thigh height. And to keep the chickens company, and the dog, and the cat ...

Paul is working really hard to get his business idea off the ground, to get it up and running. And we make sure that we take time out to celebrate each and every one of his successes, each and every milestone, the launch of his website, his first paying customer, his first sale. And Paul made the decision to set up an arrangement with a charity for the homeless so that the better his business does and the more money that it makes for him and for us, the more money that his business can give back to help young homeless people. And that seems to mean a lot to Paul these days, giving something back.

And as for me, the void that remained for a little while, after I had left behind paid employment is gradually starting to be filled with things that I find infinitely more rewarding and infinitely more valuable. I have freedom, now. I have flexibility.

My days are my own. My days are a blank sheet upon which I can write and draw and scribble and paint whatever I like. I am still doing and, more importantly, I am still *enjoying* my bits and pieces of freelance marketing work. But it's just a handful of days' work each month, just enough to pay the bills, just enough to maintain a modicum of contact with the outside world. I find that I have the time and the inclination to write. I have more time for my friends, too. Huge swathes of uninterrupted, quality time; for the friends that I have made since we moved to Ireland, for the friends that I still have in England. But, crucially, I have more time than I have ever had for myself.

I feel so much healthier than I have ever done before, I feel so much more *whole*. I feel committed to a much more holistic way of life and I feel as though that commitment has really started to pay off. I feel invigorated and I feel alive and, in so many different ways, I feel *grateful*. I feel grateful that in my seemingly tireless quest to find a solution to our involuntary childlessness, I explored so very many different avenues. Avenues that, at first, I hoped would help me to have a baby. Avenues that, in the end, turned out to have a positive impact on my entire life.

I investigated alternative therapies and I compiled a mental list of the ones that seemed right for me. I found out about the contribution that nutrition and relaxation and *happiness* could make to general well-being. I found out about the importance of being committed to a life-long journey of self-development. And so I eat well and I sleep better. I exercise most days, in a gentle and relaxing way. I swim and I walk and I practise yoga. I take time out for myself – simply to relax and to breathe, to be peaceful and to meditate. And I make sure that I do those things every single day. I make them a priority.

There are still days when I wonder if our involuntary childlessness has been a message of some sort. I am pretty sure that Paul and I would be great parents. I am pretty sure that we have something incredibly positive to offer to children. And so I wonder if maybe something *else* is meant to be for us. A different *form* of parenting, perhaps. Maybe we are meant to adopt a child, one day, or do voluntary work with kids who are in need. I know that what is meant to be will, eventually, become clear. And, until it does become clear, we are both determined to make the very most of our lives. To be happy.

And we are happy, Paul and I. In many ways we are happier, now, than we have ever been. We are *content*. And that contentment is all the more precious because there have been times when both of us were so very far from it. Over the years that we were trying for our baby, there were times when I wanted almost everything to change. I wanted to slow down time – to stop it, if I could. I wanted to stop the seconds and the hours, the days and the weeks, the months and the years from ticking past. Because every one of them that *did* tick past seemed to me to be a missed opportunity, seemed to me to be another unit of time closer to the day when there would be no more opportunities. I wanted to change my body. I wanted to change Paul's body. I wanted to change whatever it was about *both* of our bodies that was refusing to cooperate, to communicate, to let me conceive. But out of all the things in our life that I could have changed, out of all the things in our life that I *did* change, our relationship was the one thing that I clung on to.

Not being able to have babies seemed to shake the foundations of our relationship – and of our life – for a while. We seemed to have had more than our fair share of unhappy experiences, more than our fair share of painful conversations. But we lived through them. We survived them. And, our experiences have made our relationship stronger. Our experiences have brought us even closer together. And I love Paul more with every single day that passes, with every single day that we spend together.

Happy Endings?

The greatest lesson for me has been the realization that real life isn't like the movies. Sometimes there *is* no happy ever after and sometimes the happy ever after that you end up with isn't quite the one that you were expecting. The most important lesson for me has been learning to accept that.

I don't know when I *will* know that Paul and I are no longer trying to have a baby. I am no longer waiting for the day when I will wake up and think, 'Right, that's it. Today is the day. Enough is enough'.

I hear so many stories that continue to fill me with hope. A friend tells me about *her* friend. A woman who had dedicated ten years of her life to trying for a baby, who had tried everything. A woman who was close to giving up hope, and then she had gone for a scan, to check out her suitability for yet another round of IVF treatment. And she had been told that IVF *wasn't* going to be suitable for her. Because she was already eight weeks' pregnant. I read about a well known writer, a woman who was well into her forties, a woman who had thrown herself into her work because the baby thing hadn't happened for her. And then the baby thing *did* happen for her. And so I have hope but, more importantly, I have a sense of quiet and calm acceptance. I know that what will be, will be.

It used to be that having a baby – or, the prospect of *not* having a baby – was all consuming for me. It dominated my waking hours and my sleeping ones, my thoughts and my dreams. Now the baby thing is just one, very small, aspect of my life. And I find that I have developed a sense of perspective despite not getting the happy ending that I would have wished for, despite not getting the happy ending that I had always taken for granted. I don't think I'll ever feel glad that we didn't have children, Paul and I. But, most days, I do feel glad to be alive. I feel happy anyway, despite not having the children that I hoped for.

There are still days when I feel sad and I feel sorry. There are still days when I feel disappointed. There are still days when our situation seems incredibly unfair and when I rail against that unfairness. But, as time passes, those days are getting fewer and further between. And, as time passes, my outbursts are becoming less intense, less overwhelming. And, most of the time, I am happy simply to accept the card that life has dealt us, to accept the status quo.

I no longer feel the compulsion to race through life, ticking boxes – degree, job, house, husband, baby – just to make myself feel as though I am achieving something, as though I am getting on. My happiness is much less conditional these days. I read something philosophical once that really struck a chord with me. I read that although we shouldn't be happy to lose an eye, we should draw comfort from the fact that life would be possible even if we did do so. And, these days, that's exactly the way that I feel about not having had a baby.

I feel as though, finally, I have reached a place of wholeness. I have found the peace of mind that I was looking for despite not getting the outcome that I was hoping for. Sometimes I think that not having a baby was a gift – albeit a very well disguised one. Sometimes I think that not having a baby was a wonderful opportunity – a catalyst – for my own personal development and growth. Infertility has forced me to question myself and my actions and my lifestyle at an incredibly deep and fundamental level. And I don't think that I would have ever felt the need to ask those questions if I *had* been able to have children.

I am much less rigid than I ever was before. I am much more fluid. My experience of dealing with infertility has taught me that much. Sometimes there are no answers. And, sometimes, dealing with not knowing can be hard. There are times when I wish that I could look into a crystal ball to see what the future holds for us – to see if we will ever have children. But most of the time, I am happy *not* knowing. I have learnt that, sometimes, not knowing what the future holds is OK too.

Recommended Reading

Barefoot Doctor, *Return of the Urban Warrior*. Thorsons, 2001.

Alain de Botton, *The Consolations of Philosophy*. Penguin, 2001.

Richard Carlson, *Don't Sweat the Small Stuff*. Hyperion, 1997.

Daniel Goleman, *Emotional Intelligence*. Bloomsbury, 1996.

Eckhart Tolle, *The Power of Now*. Hodder and Stoughton, 2001.

Susan Jeffers, *Feel the Fear and Do It Anyway*. Rider, 1991.

Brandon Bays, *The Journey*. Element, 2003.

James van Praagh, *Meditations with ...* Rider, 2003.

Ginny Fraser, *A Mother in my Heart*. Nightlight Publishing, 2001.

Niravi B. Payne and Brenda Lane Richardson, *The Fertility Solution.* Thorsons, 2002.

Christiane Northrup, *Women's Bodies, Women's Wisdom.* Piatkus, 1995.

Michael Tierra and John Lust, *The Natural Remedy Bible.* Pocket Books, 2003.

Organizations & Additional Resources

COUNSELLING & THERAPY
British Association for Counselling and Psychotherapy
www.bacp.co.uk
BACP House, 35–37 Albert Street, Rugby, Warwickshire,
CV21 2SG

HYPNOTHERAPY
National Council for Hypnotherapy
www.hypnotherapists.org.uk
PO Box 421, Charwelton, Daventry, NN1 1AS

HOMEOPATHY
The Society of Homeopaths
www.homeopathy-soh.com
11 Brookfield, Duncan Close, Moulton Park, Northampton,
NN3 6WL

REFLEXOLOGY
Association of Reflexologists
www.reflexology.org
27 Old Gloucester Street, London, WC1N 3XX

British Reflexology Association
www.britreflex.co.uk
Monks Orchard, Whitbourne, Worcester, WR6 5RB

YOGA
British Wheel of Yoga
www.bwy.org.uk
25 Jermyn Street, Sleaford, Lincolnshire, NG34 7RU

Rusheens Yoga Centre
www.rusheensyogacentre.com
Rusheens, Ballygriffin, Kenmare, County Kerry, ROI

FERTILITY-RELATED RESOURCES
**Foresight – The Association for the Promotion of
Pre-conceptual Care**
www.foresight-preconception.org.uk
178 Hawthorn Road, West Bognor, West Sussex, PO21 2UY

Infertility Network UK
www.infertilitynetworkuk.com
Charter House, 43 St Leonards Road, Bexhill on Sea,
East Sussex, TN40 1JA

NISIG
www.infertilityireland.ie
P.O. Box 131, Togher, Co. Cork, ROI

Getting Pregnant
www.gettingpregnant.co.uk

FOOD & NUTRITION

Dr Marilyn Glenville www.marilynglenville.com

14 St Johns Road, Tunbridge Wells, TN4 9NP

Soil Association

www.soilassociation.org

Bristol House, 40–56 Victoria Street, Bristol, BS1 6BY

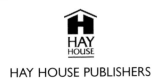

We hope you enjoyed this Hay House book.
If you would like to receive a free catalogue featuring additional
Hay House books and products, or if you would like information
about the Hay Foundation, please contact:

Hay House UK Ltd
Unit 62, Canalot Studios • 222 Kensal Rd • London W10 5BN
Tel: (44) 20 8962 1230; Fax: (44) 20 8962 1239
www.hayhouse.co.uk

****

Published and distributed in the United States of America by:
Hay House, Inc. • P.O. Box 5100 • Carlsbad, CA 92018-5100
Tel: (1) 760 431 7695 or (800) 654 5126; Fax: (1) 760 431 6948 or (800) 650 5115
www.hayhouse.com

****

Published and distributed in Australia by:
Hay House Australia Ltd • 18/36 Ralph St • Alexandria NSW 2015
Tel: (61) 2 9669 4299 • Fax: (61) 2 9669 4144
www.hayhouse.com.au

****

Published and distributed in the Republic of South Africa by:
Hay House SA (Pty) Ltd • PO Box 990 • Witkoppen 2068
Tel/Fax: (27) 11 706 6612 • orders@psdprom.co.za

****

Distributed in Canada by:
Raincoast • 9050 Shaughnessy St • Vancouver, BC V6P 6E5
Tel: (1) 604 323 7100 • Fax: (1) 604 323 2600

****

Sign up via the Hay House UK website to receive the Hay House
online newsletter and stay informed about what's going on with
your favourite authors. You'll receive bimonthly announcements
about discounts and offers, special events, product highlights,
free excerpts, giveaways, and more!

www.hayhouse.co.uk